Skinny Bitch

Book of Vegan Swaps

Also by Kim Barnouin

Skinny Bitch

Skinny Bitch in the Kitch

Skinny Bitch Bun in the Oven

Skinny Bastard

Skinny Bitchin'

Skinny Bitch: Ultimate Everyday Cookbook

Skinny Bitch Home, Beauty & Style

Skinny Bitch

Book of Vegan Swaps

Kim Barnouin

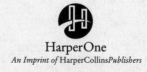

HarperOne

An Imprint of HarperCollinsPublishers

HarperOne

HarperCollins books may be purchased for educational, business, or sales promotional use. For information please write: Special Markets Department, HarperCollins Publishers, 10 East 53rd Street, New York, NY 10022.

HarperCollins website: http://www.harpercollins.com

HarperCollins®, ■®, and HarperOne™ are trademarks of HarperCollins Publishers.

FIRST EDITION

Designed by Ralph Fowler

Library of Congress Cataloging-in-Publication Data

Barnouin, Kim.
   Skinny bitch book of vegan swaps / by Kim Barnouin.
      p. cm.
   ISBN 978–0–06–210511–0
   1. Natural foods.   2. Food substitutes.   3. Food—Composition.
4. Vegetarian cooking.   I. Title.
   TX369.B365   2012
   641.3'02—dc23   2011041290

12 13 14 15 16   CJK   10 9 8 7 6 5 4 3 2 1

To my parents Linda and Rob,

I've always wanted to make you proud,

while you just cared about my happiness.

I hope I've achieved both in your eyes.

Contents

Acknowledgments

To my amazing literary agent, Laura Dail, as always, a million thanks for what you do and for all of your support.

Nancy Hancock at HarperCollins, what a pleasure it is to have you as my new editor. I am grateful for your belief in my work and me as a person. I look forward to a long future together.

Suzanne Wickham, thank you for making me look so good in the public eye—you're an amazing publicist and your efforts are so appreciated.

Suzanne Quist, I'm thankful for your hard work and expertise.

Mark Tauber, you have a badass publishing company. I am beyond excited to be under your watch.

To everyone at HarperOne who worked on this book, I'm grateful for all of your hard work and creativity. It is one fucking amazing book.

My Sanoria gang, moving to the O.C. was a new experience for me, but you made being the new kid on the block feel like an easy transition. I feel so welcome.

Sunday Long, you were my first friend here and I thank you for keeping me company in the afternoons, laughing and watching our kids play.

Jerry and Karen Prefontaine, thanks for all of the bonfires and for opening your home to Jack. And James, thank you for being such a good friend to Jack—if it wasn't for your babysitting skills, this book may have never gotten finished. (Phew.)

To Tom and Joylene Loucks, Stephane and I were never big on double dating until we met you. Thank you for always showing us a good time.

Joylene, I am so grateful to have met you and your family. You have become such a close friend and it is a friendship I will keep forever. Thank you for your heart, your laughter, and your spunk. We get each other as friends and moms, and it means a lot to me. I am so happy Jack, Brooke, and Evan love each other so much.

Carly Harrill, you are my wing woman. Thank you for being so gifted at what you do. I have much love and admiration for you.

Julie C. May, my trusted friend and business genius, I adore you.

McKenna Farver, thank you for being the best assistant ever. I really appreciate how great you were with Jack and what an enormous help you were for me while putting this book together.

Keesha Whitehurst-Fredricksen, you are the best therapist and friend a girl could have. I am one lucky bitch to have you in my life. Tons of love and laughs with you.

To Jack, what can I say about the greatest and cutest kid on earth? I love you more each day, and you never cease to amaze me with your intelligence and humor.

Stephane, my love, as always, I cherish you with all my heart and am grateful for your love and support. Thanks for staying up late at night with me to try a million different vegan products. You have a gifted palate, and a gifted heart. I love you.

And again, to all the Skinny Bitch fans, thank you for continuing to show your love and keeping the series alive. Your passion for health and all living things inspires me every day. Rock on.

Skinny **Bitch**

Book of Vegan Swaps

Introduction

So you say you're going vegan. Or at least you're going to give it a whirl. Maybe you'll just try it for a weekend. Either way, you're doing it. Yay, you.

But it's a wild, wild world out there. Beyond the meatless food trucks and vegan celebrities with live-in chefs, there's a supermarket that's ready to eat you whole, stilettos and all. Professional samplers stand behind tables shoving chicken cubes on toothpicks at you. The frozen-food aisles are full of crap I wouldn't feed to my cats. And the words "natural," "organic," and "cruelty-free" are competing for face time on packaged foods as if they were prime-time reality TV shows.

What you need, my friend, is someone who can show you the way; someone who's looking out for you.

Um, hello?! That would be me, bitch.

Let me tell you why I'm your damn knight in shining armor, princess. *Because I've been there.* I've endured months on end eating frozen bean-and-rice burritos and soup out of a can, because I had no idea what I was doing. I had decided I wasn't going to eat meat and dairy, so as long as it didn't look like it used to have legs, live on a farm, or come out of a chicken's ass, it looked good to me. But isn't that the problem? As vegans or pseudo-vegans, we tend to stuff our mouths with garbage, because we think our choices are limited. But they're not, my dear. Not even close.

So regardless of what stage you're at—going vegan cold turkey, taking the thirty-day challenge, or having been a clueless plant eater for years—this book is your supermarket bible. This is for all of you who have the compassion, decency, and dedication to make changes in your life that have an impact on our world, but just need to know what you have at your disposal and where to get it. I have done more than a year's worth of research to assemble some of the tastiest, most authentic, and healthiest products in every category from meatless BBQ wings to gelatin-free marshmallows to vegan wine and beer, so that you can have the guidance I wish I had had all along.

Let me stress one word I just mentioned: *healthy.* Aside from more pure and nourishing alternatives for traditional animal products, I take it a step farther and offer more nutritious alternatives for conventional every-day foods such as flour, tortillas, canned tomatoes, peanut butter, chips, cereal, soda, and more. Basically, this in-depth guide covers everything you will stick in your kid's mouth or put in your health-conscious pantry or refrigerator.

Here's the kick in the ass: nowadays, it's tough to tell the difference between a pineapple and a preservative. The food on our shelves is not only making us fat; it's also responsible for a number of diseases and ailments, including attention deficit disorder (ADHD), diabetes, heart disease, and even cancer. As we make transitions in our diets, we assume the responsibility for arming ourselves with the knowledge and tools to make grocery shopping a safe activity again. Because nobody is watching out for you but *you*.

I admit that not every product in this book is squeaky clean. Some still contain a few artificial ingredients I don't love. But we're human. Sometimes we need a piece of soy beef jerky or a calorie-packed salad dressing to get us through PMS or a shitty breakup. The point is to give you options. Options are key, honey. Once you know how much is out there, have the time to experiment with new products, find what your taste buds fancy, and switch things up, the rest is easy. You've eliminated your obstacles, and before you know it seitan tastes like the real thing.

Before I shut up, to make sure you are constantly entertained by this transition, I put together lists of natural-food retailers, popular airport food, and my favorite restaurants and bakeries across the country, so you'll know where to shop and where to go when you're on the road. And for those of you debating how to get started, I created a weekend vegan menu and recipes to strip away any anxiety. (I don't cope well with panic attacks.)

In a perfect world, well, *my* perfect world, ditching meat and animal products wouldn't be that tough. Healthy, meatless foods that made us feel and live better would be available in vending machines. Natural-food retailers would replace the food superstore or Starbucks on every corner. But, let's face it—the world ain't perfect. And I'll be darned, neither is the supermarket.

Until then, you're just going to have to be the chick carrying a book around the grocery store with the word *bitch* on the cover. You're welcome.

Love & Peace,
Kim

Where the Hell to Shop

It's not about who you know, but where you shop, sugar. There is no doubt that major grocery chains are getting privy to our needs with dedicated health-food sections. Hell, even superstores such as Walmart and Target carry vegan and vegetarian products that are gentle on the ole wallet nowadays.

But if you want to guarantee you will find most of the items in this book, you have to know where to push that cart. I compiled a list of retailers from all over the country for your convenience, so don't feel as though you're screwed if you don't live in a major metropolitan hub. You should be able to find one near your neighborhood.

Natural-Food Retailers

Henry's Farmers Market

A jaunt through Henry's, which has dozens of locations throughout California, will feel like you're shopping on a farm—except without the dudes in overalls. The health-food store offers a nice variety of vegan products in addition to fresh, organic produce sourced locally, whole grains in bulk bins, natural supplements, and baked goods. Everything is affordable, and you'll just want to give the staff a big hug. Henry's website even offers recipes and a blog on health and wellness. For locations, visit henrys markets.com.

Whole Foods

The Mecca of all things natural health, Whole Foods is more than just a specialty retailer for health freaks. On its floors you can find almost any product in this book, some of which belong to its private line of signature products: 365 Everyday Value. It also offers health screenings, body and personal care products, online podcasts, and a loan program for small, local food producers. My only nitpick would be that it hasn't earned the nickname "Whole Paycheck" for no reason—it tends to be on the pricier side, but you pay for the convenience of one-stop shopping. Whole Foods stores are scattered all over the United States, Canada, and the United Kingdom. For locations, visit wholefoodsmarket.com.

Sunflower Shoppe

The go-to source for natural foods and vegan and vegetarian products if you live near one in Texas. Sunflower Shoppe is family owned and operated, with one location in Forth Worth and another north of Dallas in Colleyville. Aside from the usual fresh produce, supplements, and health products, Sunflower has a café and certified nutritionists on staff. For locations, visit sunflowershoppe.com.

Sunflower Farmers Market

Not to be confused with Sunflower Shoppe, Sunflower Farmers Market is popping up in many locations with a great selection of natural and organic products for stellar prices. Visit the website to download coupons and sale flyers before hitting the aisles. There are thirty-four locations throughout Arizona, Colorado, New Mexico, Nevada, Utah, California, and Texas. For locations, visit sunflowermarkets.com.

Trader Joe's

What started as a small convenience-store chain in the 1950s is now one of the nation's beloved neighborhood markets. TJ's has a wide selection of vegetarian and vegan products, along with a private label that is hard to miss (but a bitch to find on the website). Its guidelines aren't as stringent as those of, say, Whole Foods, so read the labels to make sure a product belongs in your pantry. But the prices are awesome, and the entire staff wears Hawaiian shirts to remind you that people shouldn't take themselves too seriously. For locations, visit traderjoes.com.

Mother's Market & Kitchen

Known for catering to all dietary preferences, Mother's sticks to organic, GMO-free, vegan, vegetarian, gluten-free, low-fat, and low-sodium products. If it's on the shelves, you can guarantee it's good for you. With an on-site kitchen, deli, and juice bar, this southern California–based market also makes sure you don't walk out hungry. For locations, visit mothersmarket.com.

Bristol Farms

With an emphasis on freshness and quality, Bristol Farms appeals to any eater, including us vegans. Their stores are quaint and beautiful, with a sit-down area to enjoy some of life's simple pleasures like vegan chili or a create-your-own salad bar. The Manhattan Beach locale even offers cooking classes out of Grace-Marie's Kitchen. For locations, visit bristolfarms.com.

Kroger/Ralph's

The natural-food department at Kroger (a.k.a. Ralph's in California) is not just limited to veggie dogs and microwave meals. It may be a typical grocery store to the naked eye, but this department has a groovy selection of vegan and organic food items. For locations, visit kroger.com or ralphs.com.

Back to the Land Natural Foods

Serving Brooklyn since the early 1970s, this small natural-foods store fits a lot inside its tiny doors. It can get crowded, but expect to find organic whole foods, nutritional supplements, and body-care products all under its roof. Located at 142 7th Avenue, Brooklyn, NY 11215. For more information, visit backtothelandnaturalfoods.com.

Simple Enough Natural Foods

This one is rather undercover, but it carries hard-to-find ingredients, and it's in an accessible shopping plaza. Located at 18 Lyman Street, Westborough, MA 01581. No website, but check it out on yelp.com.

Down to Earth All Vegetarian Organic & Natural Foods Store

This Hawaiian grocer is 100 percent vegetarian and built on the ethos of respecting innocent animals. It offers a wide selection of natural and organic foods, vitamins, body-care products, and household items, with a deli that offers meatless sandwiches, smoothies, a salad bar, and eggless desserts. And this is no small-time operation—we're talking locations in Honolulu, Kailua, Pearlridge, Kahului, Hilo, and Kapolei. For locations, visit downtoearth.org.

Erewhon Natural Foods Market

Erewhon is a 12,000-square-foot grocer in Los Angeles with an excellent variety of organic produce, macrobiotics, and homeopathics. Located at 7660-B Beverly Boulevard, Los Angeles, CA 90036. For more information, visit erewhonmarket.com.

Yes! Organic Market

With seven organic markets in the greater Washington, D.C., metro area, Yes! has been supplying health-conscious consumers for three decades. The one-stop shop carries vegan and gluten-free products in addition to ayurvedic and homeopathic solutions. For locations, visit livingnaturally.com.

Marlene's Market & Deli Natural Foods

Family owned and operated in Washington, this natural-food store offers 100 percent organic produce and sustainable foods, beauty care, and household items. For locations, visit marlenesmarket.net.

Here are a handful of smaller natural-food stores across the country:

THE RAISIN RACK
Two locations, Columbus/Westerville and Canton, Ohio. For more information, visit raisinrack.com.

NEWLEAF NATURAL GROCERY
Located at 1261 West Loyola Avenue, Chicago, IL 60626. For more information, visit newleafnatural.net.

GREEN ACRES MARKET
Two locations, Kansas City and Wichita, Kansas. For more information, visit greenacres.com.

RED CLOVER MARKET
Located at 5500 Old Cheney Road, Suite 14, Lincoln, NB 68516. For more information, visit redclovermarket.wordpress.com.

Farmers Markets

Alas, no matter where home is, most towns have a local farmers market that supports community agriculture. Buy an organic pear and chances are you can shake hands with the man who grew it for you. I buy all my fruits, vegetables, jams/spreads, and flowers at my neighborhood farmers market, and it even gives me some time to get some sun. Visit localharvest.org to find a farmers market near you.

NATURAL FOODS MARKET
Located at 3211 Peoples Street, Suite 74, Johnson City, TN 37604.
For more information, visit nfmonline.com.

CHAMBERLIN'S NATURAL FOODS
Located at 430 North Orlando Avenue, Winter Park, FL 32789.
For more information, visit chamberlins.com.

Veggin' Out
A Rundown of Restaurants, Cafés, and Bakeries Serving Vegan Selections

It ain't always easy being a vegan. Okay, who am I kidding? It's a pain in the ass. (But boy is it rewarding.) Case in point: eating out. Friends are always trying to organize their birthday dinners around our eating preferences. We're often stuck ordering side dishes or indulging in yet another carb-heavy bowl of refined pasta just to pretend we're really not that difficult. As it turns out, we're pretty easy.

For all of my vegan foodies (or just foodies expanding their palates), I've compiled a list of some of the best vegan-friendly eateries across the country. Some I have had the luxury of eating at personally, and others are courtesy of Skinny Bitch fans and my fabulous Facebook friends. I even highlighted some of my favorite dishes or those that made me go ape-shit when I spotted them on the menu. Chow down, bitches.

Made for Vegans:
A Rundown of Vegan Restaurants, Grubberies, and Bakeries Across the Map

Vegan Treats [BETHLEHEM, PENNSYLVANIA]

Satisfying both ethics and your taste buds, Vegan Treats is a dessert haven of French pastries, doughnuts, brownies, cookies, cakes, and the highly sought-after Peanut Butter Bombs. The founder, Danielle Konya, has been awarded the PETA Proggy Award for Best Bakery, and she beat out fifty nonvegan bakers in PBS's Feast of Sweets (vegantreats.com).

> **KIM'S PICKS:** Vanilla Buttercream Cake, Chocolate Doughnuts, Cupcakes, Brownie Chunk Cheesecake, and the Sticky Buns.

The Loving Hut [CINCINNATI, OHIO]

A comfortable café that operates to serve every being with respect—even the trees. A sucker for sustainability, the restaurant is full of reclaimed, recycled, or yard-sale furniture and knick-knacks. The vegan cuisine errs on the healthy side, and everything is pretty affordable (thelovinghut.us/cincinnati–01).

> **KIM'S PICKS:** Happy Gyro, New Chik'n Meal, Spring Rolls, Sloppy Joes, and BBQ Hot Wings.

Sweetpea Baking Company [PORTLAND, OREGON]

On top of delectable vegan goods and pastries, Sweetpea offers homemade soups, sandwiches, bagels, breads, and espresso that follow its cruelty-free mantra. (It also caters to those with nut or gluten allergies.) As if you need an excuse, Saturday is Doughnut Day, and Sunday features an all-you-can-eat brunch (sweetpeabaking.com).

> **KIM'S PICKS:** Bananas and Cream Cake, Lemon Chiffon Cake, Black Forest Cake, Boston Cream Pie, Key Lime Cupcake, Brownie Chunk Cupcake, Raspberry Cupcake, and Coconut Cupcake.

Cakewalk Baking Company [SALT LAKE CITY, UTAH]

Although you have the right to assume that I chose this bakery because its tagline is "I Get My Protein from Cake," that is only part of it. Cake-walk satisfies the sweet tooth with a wide selection of vegan, organic, and gluten-free treats made with fair-trade ingredients. The cakes are to die for and are frosted or filled with vegan buttercream and fruit preserves. If you're one of those chicks who looks at the dessert menu before even glimpsing at the entrees, then Cakewalk might spell trouble for you (cakewalkbakingcompany.com).

> **KIM'S PICKS:** Cheesecake, Pumpkin Pie, Chocolate Cream Pie, Coconut Cream Pie, Cream Puffs, and Eclairs.

High Noon Café [JACKSON, MISSISSIPPI]

Just because a food is vegan doesn't mean it's automatically free of icky ingredients like artificial sugars, preservatives, fat, and sodium. Not the case at High Noon. The vegan and vegetarian cuisine is made from scratch every day with certified organic ingredients and no stinkin' trans fats, hydrogenated oils, MSG, or GMOs (rainbowcoop.org/cafe/Menu2011.pdf).

KIM'S PICKS: Sandwiches made with the signature Beet Burgers, especially the High Noon Reuben, Messy Mushroom, Patty Melt, and Build Your Own Grilled Cheese.

Sticky Fingers [WASHINGTON, D.C.]

Holy moly, Batman. Junk-food junkies will go nutzo for Doron Petersan's gourmet bites and sweets. With a degree in nutrition and food science, this former New Yorker has built a solid D.C. following with eats that are free of all animal products, and nut- and gluten-free options too. Did I mention that she also took the grand prize for Food Network's Cupcake Wars in 2010? How about that Sticky Fingers was voted Best Vegan Restaurant in D.C. in 2011? I'll shut my pie hole now (stickyfingersbakery.com).

KIM'S PICKS: Eggless Salad, Tuna Melt, Hot Nuggets, Red Velvet Cupcake, Cookies 'N Cake Cupcake, Almond Fudge Cupcake, Sticky Buns, and the Little Devil (a cream-filled chocolate cake sandwich).

Sprig & Vine Pure Vegetarian
[NEW HOPE, PENNSYLVANIA]

This small-town restaurant earns five stars in my book. The menu focuses on seasonal gourmet vegan cuisine made from locally grown produce. The chef behind it, Ross Olchvary, was the sous chef and chef de cuisine at Philadelphia's Horizons.

KIM'S PICKS: Housemade Doughnuts, Biscuits and Gravy, Tofu Benedict, Chocolate Pancakes, Five Spice–Blackened Tofu, and the African Groundnut Stew.

Candle Café [NEW YORK, NEW YORK]

Renowned as one of the best vegan/vegetarian restaurants in the country, Candle Café practices a farm-to-table approach, using all-organic vegan ingredients. The owners, Bart Potenza and Joy Pierson, started with a hit juice bar, vitamin shop, and café all in one on Manhattan's Upper East Side—that was until they won the lottery. They used their jackpot to open what is now New York's famed bistro and the first certified green restaurant in the city. The pair also have Candle 79, a hoity-toity restaurant in NYC with an organic wine and sake bar that has become a celebrity and influencer hot spot (candlecafe.com).

KIM'S PICKS: BBQ Tempeh and Sweet Potato Sandwich, Tuscan Seitan Parmesan Sandwich, Tuscan Lasagna, Teriyaki Seitan, Mexi-Candle Cornbread, Spring Rolls, and the Chocolate Mousse Pie.

Madeleine Bistro [TARZANA, CALIFORNIA]

Ranked as one of the Top Eight Vegetarian Restaurants in America by PETA, Madeleine's is a fancy-schmancy bistro that has won over plenty of hearts with its gourmet organic vegan cuisine. The white linen tablecloths, artsy dish presentation, and romantic lighting make it look like any other place you'd take a hot date, which, ironically, is what makes this place so different (madeleinebistro.com). How else are we gonna change the face of veganism?

(The award-winning) Beet Tartar, Mickey's D's, Chicken Fried Seitan, Classic Mac and Cheese, Cajun Gumbo, Big Mac, Chocolate Frosted Raised Donuts, and Crème Brûlée.

Millennium [SAN FRANCISCO, CALIFORNIA]

A restaurant that calls for a reservation, Millennium believes in sustainability and practices everything that goes with that, from recycling to composting to using locally sourced ingredients that are in season. The prix-fixe menu is constantly evolving, so it never gets old (millennium restaurant.com).

Kim's Picks (with the understanding that dishes are always changing): Teff Griddle Cake, Pistachio Crusted Tempeh, Huitlacoche Tamale, Stuffed Artichoke, Chocolate Almond Midnight, Peanut Butter-Chocolate Chip Bread Pudding, and Lemon Cheesecake.

Blossoming Lotus [PORTLAND, OREGON]

At the forefront of Portland's already progressive culinary scene, the Lotus is all about healthy, mouthwatering vegan fusion fare that will make you say, "Gimme more, buddy" (blpdx.com).

KIM'S PICKS: Crispy Thai BBQ Wrap, Smoked Maple Tempeh, Spicy BBQ Sandwich, Southwest Bowl, Creole Bowl, and the Softy Shake (made with their signature soft serve).

Flying Apron [SEATTLE, WASHINGTON]

Located in the heart of Seattle's Fremont neighborhood, the Flying Apron is one of the few organic vegan bakeries in the area that does without the gluten and the wheat (flyingapron.com).

> **KIM'S PICKS:** Apple Pie Filling, Berry Scone, Dark Chocolate Cupcake with Chocolate Frosting, Shepherd's Pie, Personal Pizza, and Macaroni and Chez.

Karyn's on Green [CHICAGO, ILLINOIS]

If you're looking to get laid, this contemporary hot spot attracts the crème de la crème of Chicago with vegan food that oozes style. Think minimalistic with a remarkable view and soft, sexy lighting. The menu revolves around modern American cuisine with the spotlight on presentation (karynson green.com).

> **KIM'S PICKS:** French Toast, Creamy Grits, Potato Leek Soup, Crab Sliders, Buffalo Chicken Pita, Seared Tofu Gumbo, Chocolate Terrine, and Sweet Potato Pie with Marshmallow Cream.

Chrissie Hynde's VegiTerranean [AKRON, OHIO]

If you're a vegan with worldly flair, VegiTerranean offers just what it sounds like: plant-based Italian and Mediterranean cuisine. The brainchild of Ohio native and lead singer of the rock band The Pretenders, this upscale joint has an industrial, warehouse atmosphere and a good crowd (thevegi terranean.com).

> **KIM'S PICKS:** Tuscan Grilled Eggplant Parmesan over Crispy Gnocchi Arrabbiata and Baby Arugula, "Chicken" Picatta, Fresh

Spinach Fettuccini with Wild Mushrooms and Roasted Artichoke Madeira Thyme Cashew Cream Sauce, Rubber City Melt, and Biker Burger.

Herbivore: The Earthly Grill

Serving up an international vegan menu, this award-winning grill has taken home its fair share of trophies in the Bay Area—now with three locations. The setting is comfortable and casual for lunch or a relaxing dinner with friends (herbivorerestaurant.com).

KIM'S PICKS: Basil Pesto Scrambled Tofu, Doughnuts, "Sausage" Biscuit, Crepes, Soft Tacos, Coconut Noodle Soup, Moussaka, Pad Thai, Ravioli, and Kung Pao.

Yuan Fu Vegetarian [ROCKVILLE, MARYLAND]

From the looks of it, you'd think you were entering a traditional Chinese restaurant. But this isn't your everyday soy-sauce and chopsticks establishment. The entire menu is plant-based, despite the traditional animal names. Yuan Fu uses no MSG and even offers a nonfat menu for those watching their weight (yuanfuvegetarian.com).

KIM'S PICKS: Kung Pao Chicken with Portabella Mushrooms, Veggie Duck with Chinese Broccoli, Fried Tofu with Basil and Ginger in Hot Pot, Sesame Chicken with Broccoli, Moo Shi Pork, Beef with Snow Peas, and Steamed Dumplings.

Native Foods Café

Yet another southern California chain that has changed the way people look at vegan food, Native Café caters to the plant eater with healthy, balanced, and nutritious fare. The restaurant's founder, Chef Tanya (she's like Prince, no need for a last name), makes everything from scratch on a daily basis. Simply delicious (nativefoods.com).

> **KIM'S PICKS:** Native Nachos, Spicy Buffalo Wings, Super Italian Meatball Sub, Oklahoma Bacon Cheeseburger, Chicken Run Ranch Burger, PB&J Cheesecake (my sweet husband has ordered a whole cheesecake for quite a few of my birthdays), and Chocolate Love Pie.

Sublime [FT. LAUDERDALE, FLORIDA]

Located in my hometown, Sublime is just that . . . sublime. Its vegan menu features natural and organic foods and spirits with a worldly flare, while the lively atmosphere appeals to all senses. And don't be surprised if you end up rubbing elbows with a celeb—Paul McCartney, Pamela Anderson, and Alec Baldwin are just a few of the pretty faces that have been spotted eating there (sublimerestaurant.com).

> **KIM'S PICKS:** Fire-Roasted Artichoke, Broccoli Cheddar Quiche, Shepherdless Pie, Mac and Cheese, Kale Salad, Chocolate Nirvana, Coconut Cake, and Key Lime Cheesecake.

The Veggie Grill

[SEVEN LOCATIONS IN SOUTHERN CALIFORNIA]

In the early 1980s, the twelve-year Oxford Vegetarian Study followed eleven thousand subjects to assess the differences between vegans and meat eaters. A crazy finding? The death rate from heart disease was lower in plant eaters than meat eaters.

The Veggie Grill serves, hands down, the most ridiculously tasty fast food–style vegan food you will ever sink your teeth into. I waited on one of the owners, Kevin Boylan, when I was a waitress in Los Angeles, and he had recently read *Skinny Bitch.* He was getting ready to launch a veggie chain, and I remember his passion for bringing good, healthy vegan sandwiches and burgers to the restaurant industry. I later met his partner, T. K. Pillan, and I must say, I couldn't be more excited that their chain is taking off. Though they are currently only in SoCal, expect to see the Veggie Grill in a neighborhood near you very soon. P.S.: They also have a kid's menu (veggiegrill.com).

KIM'S PICKS: Chill Out Wings, Uptown Nachos, Mac-n-Cheese, Thai Chicken Salad, Chop-Chop Chef Salad, Chickin' Caesar Wrap, Santa Fe Crispy Chickin', Carne Asada, and Chocolate Pudding.

Veggin' Out at Popular Restaurant Chains

Major corporations and restaurateurs know we're here, and they know it would be stupid not to get us in their doors. Now I'm not going to bite my tongue here—a handful of these chains are part of the reason why America's known as fat, but every once in a while we all need to break the rules.

Subway

Try the Veggie Delight Salad, which also comes as a sub or wrap. The vegan breads include the Italian White, Roasted Garlic, Ciabatta, and the Hearty Italian (subway.com).

Baskin-Robbins

Not all thirty-one flavors make the cut, but the key is to stick with sorbets. Pack that waffle cone with one of these: Tropical Ice, Lemon Sorbet, Lime Daiquiri Ice, Strawberry Sorbet, or Pink Grapefruit Sorbet (baskin robbins.com).

Au Bon Pain

This chain is scattered all over the country, along with pop-up restaurants in many airports. Though you want to check its website for updated menu changes and food ingredients, Au Bon Pain is an equal-opportunity eatery. It offers a vegan soup almost daily and carries six vegan salad dressings so you can customize to any salad. If you're lunchin', the Mayan Chicken Harvest Rice Bowl with Brown Rice can be made without the chicken. Other vegan favorites are the Oatmeal, Hummus, and Olives on Sun-Dried Tomato Bread and bagels in Cinnamon Raisin, Plain, Poppy Seed, Sesame Seed, or Whole Wheat Skinny (aubonpain.com).

Chipotle Mexican Grill

Known for sourcing humanely raised meat, this healthier fast food–style chain does think outside the factory farm. You can customize any burrito, bowl, taco, or salad to be 100 percent vegan. (Just stick with the black beans, since the pintos are made with lard or bacon.) Other items that get the vegan green light? The steamed Cilantro-Lime Rice, guacamole, romaine lettuce, fajita vegetables sautéed in soybean oil, and a variety of salsas (chipotle.com).

P. F. Chang's China Bistro

Thanks to the fact that vegans have big mouths and aren't afraid to demand meatless cuisine from P. F. Chang's management, the Chinese chain has a decent selection of vegan options. Plus, the kitchen will convert any meat dish into a vegan one by substituting tofu, five-spice pressed bean curd, and vegetarian "oyster" sauce. Some of my favorites are the Vegetarian Lettuce Wraps, Kung Pao Bean Curd, Coconut Curry Vegetables, and Chang's Bean Curd (pfchangs.com).

Johnny Rockets

True, your chances are about 99 percent that you'll be sitting next to some obnoxious dude chowing down on a meat patty, but Johnny Rockets is

Is there anyplace you're pissed I left out? Well, don't be shy . . . let me know. Submit your favorite vegan restaurants for possible feature on our online spin-off, healthybitchdaily.com, by e-mailing info@healthybitchdaily.com.

savvy about vegans' need for a classic hamburger sans the cruelty. Try the Soy Boca Burger, a.k.a. the Streamliner, with grilled onions, lettuce, tomato, pickles, and mustard. There's been some controversy over whether the fries are cooked in vegetable oil or animal fat, but it's best to ask the manager. With that said, the corporate office says it always urges the use of vegetable oil. Hey, it's nice to be able to visit a burger joint and not sit there and starve (johnnyrockets.com).

Romano's Macaroni Grill

A regular in shopping plazas across the country, Macaroni Grill offers a special section on its website for vegetarian options, but, as with all non-vegan restaurants, you should check the menu in your neighborhood. You can always call ahead or pull the manager aside and use your charm to make vegan requests. Some of the vegan alternatives include the Tomato Bruschetta without cheese, Peasant Bread, Mediterranean Olives, Warm Spinach Salad with Roasted Garlic, Fresh Lemon, and Olive Oil, Capellini Pomodoro, and the Create Your Own Pasta. Any pasta works, but for sauces and toppings you'll want to stick with the arrabbiata, tomato basil, fresh broccoli, fresh mushrooms, fresh spinach, grape tomatoes, roasted garlic, and sun-dried tomatoes (macaronigrill.com).

Taco Bell

Although Taco Bell isn't my first choice, it does have vegan options. Try the Bean Burrito (without cheese), Bean Tostada (without cheese), Nachos (without cheese), Mexican Rice (without cheese), Seven Layer Burrito (without sour cream or cheese), Taco Salad (without meat, sour cream, and cheese), or the Veggie Fajita Wrap (tacobell.com).

Olive Garden

The restaurant chain that takes the cake for the cheesiest commercials doesn't make everything so cheesy. Try the house garden salad with oil and vinegar dressing (skip the croutons), steamed veggies, minestrone soup, or the Capellini Pomodoro. Top any pasta—angel hair, fettuccine, linguine, penne, shells, or spaghetti—with marinara or tomato sauce, and you've got yourself some vegan carbs (olivegarden.com).

California Pizza Kitchen

Arguably one of my favorite places on this planet, CPK is perfect for a sit-down meal or one on the go. Vegans do not starve or make sacrifices at this establishment. Try the Asparagus and Arugula Salad (without cheese), White Corn Guacamole, Lettuce Wraps with Chinese Vegetables, Tuscan Hummus, Dakota Smashed Pea and Barley Soup, Chinese Chicken Salad (without chicken or wontons), Field Greens Salad (without Dijon Balsamic or candied walnuts), Tomato Basil Spaghettini, or the Vegetarian Pizza with Japanese Eggplant (thin crust, without cheese; cpk.com).

CHAPTER

3

What to Eat at the Airport

Y ou're about to board a three-hour flight, and your stomach won't
shut up. You need to put something in that belly, but a quick scan
of the airport cafeteria tells you that you have two options: (a) chug
a few beers to fill 'er up, or (b) chew on your arm on the plane.

Though those may sound like your only options, airports aren't the fast-
food paradise they once were. Use this list to prepare before the next time
you fly the unfriendly skies.

Starbucks

Grab the Starbucks Perfect Oatmeal made with whole-grain oats, a hearty
filling breakfast.

California Pizza Kitchen

Try the Grilled Vegetable Salad with Thai Peanut Dressing. Fresh and tasty, the dressing really steals the show here.

Au Bon Pain

The soups are fantastic, including French Moroccan Tomato Lentil Soup, Black Bean Soup, Curried Rice and Lentil Soup, Tuscan White Bean, Vegetarian Chili, and Vegetarian Lentil Soup.

— THE SKINNY —

Airplane Food

Call the airline at least twenty-four hours prior to boarding to label yourself as a "vegan" if a meal is served on your flight. Be specific and ask what your options are; otherwise you may get fish or a cheese sandwich. Don't wait until you are boarding, because chances are you'll be shit out of luck.

Wolfgang Puck Express

Italian food has my name written all over it, but I can't help but get giddy when I see a Wolfgang Puck Express at an airport I'm passing through. The angel hair pasta with fresh tomato, basil, and garlic is to die for. Just do everyone a favor and pop a mint before boarding.

Smoothie King

Instead of getting hopped up on soda or coffee, order the Pomegranate Punch, which is more refreshing and healthy. The smoothie contains pomegranate juice, bananas, blueberries, apple juice, and soy protein. Leave out the turbinado sugar, which will reduce the amount of sugar and calories. You don't need it—fruit is sweet enough on its own.

Sbarro

This pizza haven offers a fancy selection of salads when you're in the mood for something light and tasty. I skip the dressings altogether and use oil and vinegar. My top picks are the Tomato and Cucumber Salad, Garden Fresh Salad, String Bean and Cherry Tomato Salad, and the Greek Salad with no cheese.

Weekend Vegan

Maybe you're not ready to make the plunge yet. You saw some animal cruelty documentary that got you thinking, but you want to take things slow if you're going to give up filet mignon and bacon. You used to like the movie *Babe*, but although you're not bawling your eyes out over it, now you do tend to tear up.

It's perfectly okay if you want to inch your way into a new way of eating—everybody's doing it. The movement started with meatless Mondays, and naturally the next logical step in this vegan*ish* evolution is the "weekend vegan." This is usually someone who doesn't mind experimenting on the weekend, but wants to avoid the weekday guilt when there are more important things to worry about like deadlines and shuttling your little monsters to soccer practice. Some of you will eventually make the full transition, but the rest of you may feel totally comfortable lessening your meat intake and thereby lowering your environmental impact. Hey, nobody's judging—except all your close friends, who secretly love to see you fail—so why not give it a shot, right?

To get you started, I created a healthy Skinny Bitch menu that will help alleviate some of the pressures of being a clueless plant eater . . . for at least one weekend:

Friday

DINNER: Crock Pot Shepherd's Pie, with veggie broth, mushrooms, potatoes, carrots, celery, herbs, and ground seitan, tempeh, or lentils. Serve with a side garden salad.

Saturday

BREAKFAST: Blueberry Pancakes with 100 percent pure maple syrup and soy sausage links. Serve with a cup of green tea and cantaloupe slices.

LUNCH: Burrito: a whole-grain tortilla filled with black beans, diced tomatoes, diced avocado, cooked scrambled tofu with taco seasoning, shredded vegan cheddar cheese, and a dab of soy sour cream. Serve with a side of fresh berries.

DINNER: Pepperoni veggie pizza, with homemade dough, Muir Glen Organic Pizza Sauce, Lightlife Smart Deli Pepperoni slices, shredded mozzarella cheese, sliced mushrooms, and chopped onions. Serve with a side garden salad.

Sunday

BREAKFAST: Breakfast bowl made of oatmeal with almond milk (or any milk substitute), a splash of brown rice syrup, sunflower seeds, sliced strawberries and banana cream on top (freeze banana slices in a zip-top bag overnight; in the morning blend frozen banana slices in a food processor until creamy).

LUNCH: Coconut curry tempeh and brown rice veggie bowl made with Turtle Island Foods Coconut Curry Tempeh Strips, Uncle Ben's Whole Grain Fast and Natural Instant Brown Rice, and sautéed veggies of your choice topped with Mike's Organic Curry Love Sauce.

DINNER: Cajun Seitan Gumbo, made with Soyrizo sausage, vegan chicken, canned tomatoes, veggie broth, onions, veggies, cumin, and chili powder. Serve on a bed of brown rice with a side garden salad.

fat
fact

We're getting bigger. Today, more than 7.3 million Americans are vegetarians and 1 million are vegans. Thanks to us, the number of land animals killed and eaten for food decreased by 300 million from 2008 to 2009.

Weekend Snacks

Avoid the urge to succumb to carnivorous temptations by keeping snacks in proximity. Here are a few things I like to keep stocked in my purse and in the pantry to use as quick fixes in between meals:

- Cornbread muffins

- Banana nut bread

- Seasonal fruit salad

- Trail mix

- Energy bars

- Hot cereal to go: Dr. McDougall's hot cereal cups (see "Cereal")

- Whole-grain English muffins with sliced tomato, sliced avocado, and shredded cheese (just heat in the broiler or oven until warm)

- Unbuttered popcorn lightly sprayed with Bragg's Liquid Amino Acids (see "Soy Sauce")

- Chips and salsa (or guacamole)

- Whole-grain pretzels

- Soy, coconut, or rice milk yogurt with sliced fruit

- Nachos with soy cheese

- So Delicious Coconut Yogurt Smoothie (see "Yogurt")

- Crackers with slices of cheese

- Pirates Booty, Veggie (see "Chips and Crackers")

- Original Tings Corn Sticks (see "Chips and Crackers")

- Soymilk drink boxes, vanilla or chocolate (see "Milk")

- Applesauce

- ZenSoy organic soy pudding (see "Pudding and Gels")

- Peanut butter and jelly sandwich

- Hummus with raw veggies and pita bread

- Dr. McDougall's baked ramen noodles soup cups

(see "Ramen Noodles")

- Soy jerky (see "Beef Jerky")

- Flavored firm tofu in smoked BBQ, teriyaki, or pineapple teriyaki sauce, cut into cubes (see "Tofu")

- Whole-grain bagels with Earth Balance butter, peanut butter, and bananas

- Graham crackers

- Baked potato with steamed veggies and Earth Balance

- Oven-roasted rosemary sweet potato fries

- Pita chips

- Baked chickpeas with cinnamon and sugar

- Sliced avocado and tomatoes drizzled with olive oil and sea salt

- Avocado and black-bean salsa with tortilla chips

- Celery with peanut butter

My Vegan Rolodex:
A Few of My Favorite Plant-Based Recipes

With nearly ten years under my belt as a vegan, I have meatless and dairy-free recipes coming out of my ass. But there are a few dozen I keep within a close distance for any and all occasions. Some are simple. Some are not for the faint of heart. And some are just to cheer me up when I want to strangle someone. Whatever makes them particularly special, they earn their own category in my recipe Rolodex.

Blueberry and Lemon Cream Parfait

Easy to prepare, light, and refreshing. This parfait is a divine treat, but who says you can't have dessert for breakfast? Not me.

Yield: 4 servings

6 ounces soy or rice milk vanilla yogurt
4 ounces cream cheese alternative (Tofutti or Follow Your
  Heart brand)
1 teaspoon raw agave nectar (or maple syrup)
1 teaspoon lemon zest, freshly grated
1 teaspoon ground flax or chia seeds
3 cups fresh blueberries

In a medium bowl, combine the yogurt, cream cheese, and agave nectar. Beat on high speed with an electric mixer until the mixture is light and creamy. Stir in the lemon zest and the seeds. Layer the cream and blueberries in tall cups or dessert dishes. Eat immediately, or cover and refrigerate.

Pizza Dough

I love to see the look on people's faces when I tell them I still eat pizza. They just can't understand how that's even possible. Well, it's more than possible, and yes, it's delicious. You can add any topping, and thanks to a new influx of vegan cheeses, you get an ooey, gooey, cheesy pizza. This dough recipe can be used for making calzones or potpies as well.

Yield: 8 slices

1 cup warm water
½ teaspoon active dry yeast
½ teaspoon evaporated cane sugar
½ teaspoon sea salt
2 tablespoons olive oil, divided
2 cups unbleached white pastry flour
1 cup unbleached whole-wheat flour

Preheat the oven to 400 degrees F. In a large mixing bowl, combine the water, yeast, and sugar and let sit until the mixture begins to bubble, about 5 minutes. Add the salt and 1 tablespoon of the olive oil to the yeast mixture. Slowly add the pastry flour. When the dough starts to thicken, use your hands to mix in the wheat flour and knead until smooth. Place the dough in a large oven-safe bowl that has been lightly oiled and cover with plastic wrap.

Set the dough in the oven (not turned on) until doubled in size, about an hour. When the dough has expanded, place on a floured cutting board or a flat surface and roll out the dough to desired size or shape. Transfer the dough to an oiled baking sheet. Top with desired ingredients and bake 15 or 20 minutes.

Toppings:

Muir Glen or Eden Organic pizza sauce

Shredded mozzarella vegan cheese (try Daiya or Follow Your Heart)

Your choice of veggies: sliced mushrooms, onions, olives, green peppers, arugula, artichokes, tomatoes, or pineapple

Vegan pepperoni slices

Chopped vegan Italian sausage

Chopped vegan ham

Chopped fresh basil

Dried or chopped fresh oregano

Pesto sauce instead of tomato sauce

Pistachio and Cardamom Biscotti

I love biscotti—such a nice combination of sweet and crunchy. I made a plain version for my son when he was teething and quickly decided I wanted a grown-up version for myself. So this recipe was born from my little one's baby biscotti. Great for dipping in hot cocoa or tea.

Yield: 16 biscotti

2 cups all-purpose flour
2 teaspoons baking powder
2 tablespoons cornstarch
1 teaspoon ground cardamom
¼ teaspoon salt
½ cup silken tofu
½ cup Earth Balance butter
2 teaspoons pure vanilla extract
¾ cup evaporated cane juice crystals
1 cup pistachios, chopped

Preheat the oven to 350 degrees F. In a large bowl, whisk together the flour, baking powder, cornstarch, cardamom, and salt. Set aside. In a food processor or blender, process the tofu until creamy. Then add the butter and vanilla extract and blend until creamy. Add the sugar and pulse until mixed well. Pour the tofu batter into the flour mixture and stir until well combined and a dough starts to form. Add the pistachios and mix well.

On a lightly floured surface, roll the dough into two logs about 10 inches long and 2 to 3 inches wide. Place on a lightly greased baking sheet and bake for 30 minutes, until firm to the touch. Remove from the oven and place on a wire rack; let cool for 15 minutes.

Reduce the oven temperature to 300 degrees F. Transfer the log to a cutting board and, using a serrated knife, cut the log into slices about ½ inch thick on the diagonal. Arrange evenly on baking sheet. Bake for 10 minutes; turn over and bake for an additional 10 minutes. Let cool on a wire rack.

Deb's Chili

My dear friend Carly nabbed this chili recipe from her mom, and everyone loves it. I can never pass up a chili. It's so easy to make, and it's loaded with protein and fiber. You can also make it ahead of time in a slow cooker, while you're at work or running daily errands. Whenever I make this recipe, I wrap it in a burrito and have it for breakfast. Don't let anyone tell you it's just for dinner.

Yield: 6 servings

2 tablespoons grapeseed oil
1 medium onion, finely diced
1 (4-ounce) can green chilies, diced
1 envelope taco seasoning
1 (28-ounce) can tomatoes, diced
1 (15-ounce) can kidney beans, drained and rinsed
1 (15-ounce) can black beans, drained and rinsed

½ cup salsa
⅔ cup vegan cheddar cheese, shredded
¼ cup vegan sour cream

In a large saucepan, heat the oil over medium heat and sauté the onions until soft, about 5 minutes. Stir in the chilies, taco seasoning, tomatoes, kidney beans, and black beans. Let the mixture simmer for about 15 to 20 minutes. Serve with salsa, cheese, and sour cream.

Corn, Asparagus, and Fresh Risotto

Risotto is one of those dishes that are so hearty and filling. Just add some veggies in there, and it's healthy too. Don't be intimidated by the thought of cooking risotto—work up some balls. It's not too difficult and doesn't take as long to cook as most people think. Also, risotto can be eaten as is or with a protein such as sautéed seitan or tempeh strips. Mmmm . . .

Yield: 8 servings

6½ cups vegetable broth
3 ears of fresh white or yellow corn, husks and silk removed
2 to 3 tablespoons grapeseed oil
1 small onion, finely chopped
⅓ cup (about 2) shallots, finely chopped
1½ cups asparagus, cut into 1-inch pieces
2 cloves of garlic, minced
1½ cups arborio rice
⅓ to ½ cup white wine

1 cup freshly shelled peas (frozen can be used too)
2 ounces vegan parmesan

In a large pot, bring the vegetable broth to a simmer on medium-low heat; then cover, and continue simmering on low heat. Place the corn in a pot of boiling water, cover and cook for 6 minutes. Drain and set aside until cool enough to handle. Remove the kernels from the cob by holding cob upright over a plate. Take a sharp knife and slice down each side, removing the kernels and the juice. Set the corn aside and put the cobs into the vegetable broth to flavor it.

In a large saucepan, heat the grapeseed oil over medium heat. Add the onion and shallots and cook until softened and translucent, about 5 minutes. Add the asparagus and sauté until well combined with onions and oil. Add the garlic and sauté for 1 minute, being careful not

— THE SKINNY —

Risotto

The trick to a kick-ass risotto is to flavor your stock with the main ingredient you're using in the risotto. That way, the finished risotto has many layers of the flavor. In this recipe, we've added the corn-cobs to the broth, which will add another layer of corn flavor on top of the one you get when you take a bite of the corn in the recipe.

to burn the garlic. Add the rice and stir, coating the grains with oil, for 2 minutes. Add the wine and stir until the wine is absorbed. Add 1 cup of the warm broth and stir constantly with a wooden spoon, until nearly absorbed. Continue adding the broth ½ cup at a time, stirring frequently and letting each addition be absorbed before adding the next, until rice is just tender and creamy looking. The risotto is done when the rice is al dente and suspended in a thick, creamy sauce, about 30 to 40 minutes.

While the risotto is cooking, blanch the peas in boiling salted water for 30 seconds. Drain. Stir the corn, asparagus, peas, and cheese into the rice. Season with salt and pepper. If the risotto is too thick, add a little more broth until it becomes creamy.

Mint Chocolate Whoopee Pie

Something about mint and chocolate together drives me wild. It reminds me of trips to Baskin-Robbins as a kid, a reward for scoring high on my report card. Mint chocolate chip was always my favorite flavor. And since you won't catch me hanging out at 31 Flavors much anymore, this pie is my treat for the whole fam. Who needs a stinkin' report card?!

Yield: 12 pies

1 cup almond milk
1 teaspoon apple cider vinegar
2 cups all-purpose flour
½ cup cocoa powder
1 teaspoon baking soda

½ teaspoon baking powder

1 tablespoon arrowroot powder (or cornstarch)

¼ teaspoon salt

½ cup Earth Balance nondairy butter, room temperature

½ cup dark brown sugar

½ cup evaporated cane juice crystals

1 teaspoon vanilla extract

½ teaspoon almond extract

FOR THE FILLING:

½ cup nonhydrogenated shortening

½ cup Earth Balance nondairy butter, room temperature

3½ cups confectioners' sugar, sifted

1½ teaspoons peppermint extract

¼ cup almond milk

Heat the oven to 375 degrees F. In a small bowl, whisk together the almond milk and vinegar and set aside (it will curdle a little; it's supposed to do that). In a separate bowl, sift together the flour, cocoa powder, baking soda, baking powder, arrowroot, and salt.

In a large bowl, beat together the butter and sugars on low speed until creamy, about 3 minutes. Increase the speed to medium and beat until fluffy and smooth, about 3 minutes. Add half of the flour mixture and half of the almond milk mixture to the batter and beat on low speed until just incorporated. Add the remaining flour mixture and almond milk mixture and beat until thoroughly combined.

Drop the batter by tablespoonfuls onto a lightly greased baking sheet, spacing them about 3 inches apart. Bake for about 10 minutes. Remove from the oven and let the cakes cool on the sheet for about 5 minutes before placing them on a rack to cool completely.

For the filling:

In a large bowl, beat the shortening and Earth Balance together until well combined. Add the confectioners' sugar and beat on medium speed for about 3 minutes. Add the peppermint extract and almond milk and beat for another 5 to 7 minutes, until fluffy.

Slice each of the cakes in half horizontally and fill with peppermint cream filling.

Ratatouille

Ratatouille is a classic French dish, and since I happen to have a French lover (okay, he's my husband), I thought it would be nice to add a little European flair to the recipes. Traditionally more time, energy, and ingredients go into making this dish, but I wanted to make it easy and semiquick for when you want gourmet in a hurry. You can eat it hot or cold (we almost prefer it cold). I like it served with a sliced slab of fried tofu, rice, or some crusty French bread.

Yield: 6 servings

¼ cup grapeseed oil
1 medium yellow onion, chopped
6 garlic cloves, peeled and smashed
1 red bell pepper, cut in large cubes
1 large eggplant, cut in large cubes
2 medium zucchini, cut in large cubes
2 roma tomatoes, cut in large cubes

1 tablespoon fresh thyme, minced
1 bay leaf

In a large sauté pan, heat the oil over medium heat. Add the onions and sauté until soft, about 5 minutes. Add the garlic and cook another 1 minute (make sure not to burn the garlic). Add the red bell pepper and sauté about 2 minutes. Add the eggplant, stir well to coat in the oil, and sauté about 2 minutes. Then add the zucchini and tomatoes and mix well with the other veggies. Season with salt and pepper to taste. Sprinkle the thyme on top and add the bay leaf. Cover and simmer on low until vegetables are soft, about 30 minutes.

Cherry Jam-Filled Muffins

I'm kind of a dessert whore. I love jelly doughnuts, and I'm obsessed with cupcakes, so here is the best of both worlds in a superdelicious fluffy jelly muffin. Here the almond extract and cherry jam really complement one another. This is great for an anytime treat or snack.

Yield: 12 muffins

1 cup almond milk (or any milk alternative)
1 teaspoon apple cider vinegar
1¾ cup all-purpose unbleached flour (or whole-wheat flour)
¾ teaspoon baking powder
½ teaspoon baking soda
½ teaspoon salt
½ cup evaporated cane juice crystals

½ cup light brown sugar

½ cup grapeseed oil

2 teaspoons almond extract

1 teaspoon vanilla extract

4 tablespoons cherry jam

Preheat the oven to 325 degrees F. In a large bowl, add the almond milk and apple cider vinegar; set aside (it will curdle a little bit; it's supposed to do that). In a separate medium bowl, add the flour, baking powder, baking soda, and salt; mix well. Add the sugars, oil, and extracts to the large bowl of almond milk and apple cider vinegar, and whisk until well combined. Add the flour mixture to the liquid and continue to whisk until smooth and batter has no lumps. Spoon into lined muffin tins, about two-thirds full. With a small teaspoon, place about 1 teaspoon of cherry jam in the center of the muffin batter and press lightly with the spoon. Bake for 20 minutes.

Peanut Seitan Noodles

This is one of my favorite dishes, hands down. You can eat it hot for dinner and cold the next day for lunch. It is that versatile and flavorful. On top of that, it's quick, healthy, and easy to make. The kids will even love it—just change up the pasta shapes for more fun and variety.

Yield: 6 servings

8 ounces whole-wheat spaghetti

1 cup snow peas

2 tablespoons sesame oil

1 cup seitan, cubed

½ cup carrots, shredded

¼ cup cucumbers, chopped (English or Persian)

¼ cup unsalted peanuts, chopped

1 tablespoon sesame seeds

1 scallion, thinly sliced

FOR THE DRESSING:

½ cup creamy peanut butter

1 tablespoon brown sugar

2 tablespoons soy sauce or Braggs Liquid Aminos

1 tablespoon sesame oil

1 tablespoon rice vinegar

Cook the pasta according to package directions; add the snow peas to the boiling water about 1 minute before pasta is about cooked, then drain. Heat the oil in a medium skillet and add the seitan; sauté over medium heat for about 5 minutes.

In a large bowl, mix together all the ingredients for the dressing and whisk until well combined and smooth. Add the noodles, snow peas, carrots, cucumbers, and peanuts to the dressing and toss until ingredients are well coated. When done, add the seitan to the noodle mixture. Top each serving with sesame seeds and scallions.

Not-Pork Stew

Obviously I live in a no-pork household. The only piggies in my home are on my kid's feet (okay, cheesy mom's humor). This stew gives me a piece of my nonvegan days back without the guilt. And it's take-a-hot-shower-to-cool-down good.

Yield: 6 servings

2 to 3 tablespoons of grapeseed oil (enough to coat the bottom of the pan)

2 cups Match Ground Pork, shaped into meatballs

6 small new potatoes, cut into quarters

1 package (9 ounces) frozen cut green beans, or ½ pound fresh green beans, trimmed and cut into 1-inch pieces

3 carrots, peeled and cut into ½-inch-thick pieces

1 large onion, chopped

2 cups low-sodium vegetable broth

1 tablespoon vegan Worcestershire sauce

1½ teaspoons dried Italian seasoning

½ teaspoon salt

¼ teaspoon black pepper

½ cup vegan sour cream

1 tablespoon cornstarch

1 teaspoon ground sweet paprika

In a 4-quart pot, heat the oil over medium-high heat, then add the ground pork meatballs. Cook for about 5 minutes, stirring frequently.

fat fact

Don't have a panic attack if you can't find paprika. It is sold at most natural health-food stores, but you can always buy it at amazon.com.

Remove the "pork" from the pan with a slotted spoon and set aside on a dish. Add the potatoes, green beans, carrots, onion, broth, Worcestershire sauce, Italian seasoning, salt, and pepper to the pot. Bring to a boil; reduce heat and simmer covered, about 15 minutes, or until vegetables are tender. Add the "pork" back in and simmer another 5 minutes.

In a small bowl, whisk together the sour cream, cornstarch, and paprika. Add to the pot of vegetables and mix well, cooking an additional 5 minutes.

Ten Habits
of a Healthy Vegan

There is a fallacy that because you're not shredding a chicken leg with your teeth or attending cheese festivals, you're eating much better. Listen here, dollface. Your sacrifice is based on compassion, preference, or alleviating gassiness or irritable bowel movements (sorry, had to go there). But ditching meat and dairy doesn't make you a healthy broad, unless you're putting the right things into your body. Processed fake bacon in the morning, chips and salsa for lunch, and Hot Tamales for dinner are far from what I call a healthy dietary regimen. Set some goals and follow these tips to become the poster child for veganism.

1. TAKE A VEGAN COOKING CLASS. Watch, and you shall learn. Gather a group of girlfriends or, better yet, a romantic partner and attend a vegan cooking class to get savvy on cooking with herbs, spices, and vegetables. Sure, you're only paying to make a few dishes under the guidance of an instructor, but what cooking classes are great for is expanding your creativity. Don't be a sissy; open your horizons.

If classes aren't your style, watch cooking shows. They are a great resource for learning how to cook or gaining some fresh ideas on what to cook. I love the Food Network. I watch what the cooks make and put my twist on it to veganize the recipes. I've learned so much from that network that I pretend I'm hosting my own show when I'm making dinner sometimes. My son looks at me weird, but one day he'll be a great cook because of my fabulous instruction!

2. KEEP IT WHOLESOME. Your diet should focus on whole grains, legumes, nuts, seeds, fruit, and veggies. If that's tough to remember, your food should be in its most natural state—the less processed the better.

3. CARRY HEALTHY SNACKS AROUND. Keep healthy bites on hand at all times to avoid falling off the healthy vegan wagon. Nutrition bars, trail mix, whole-grain crackers, or sliced veggies and fruit are always winners. I even take a small cooler for cold things in the car when I'm going to be out and about most of the day.

4. SET REALISTIC GOALS WHEN MAKING THE TRANSITION. Dropping meat and dairy cold turkey might not be the best way to ensure long-term success when adapting to a vegan diet. Gradually replace certain foods in your diet. I always recommend finding a nondairy alternative for cow's milk first; then move on to a cheese substitute, and then cut white, refined sugar out of your diet for a healthier sweetener alternative such as evaporated cane sugar or stevia. Focus on meat last if you have carnivorous tendencies, because that will be the toughest. Make a change once a week or once a month—whatever fits within your lifestyle and nutrition goals.

5. READ FOOD LABELS. Does it take you a few minutes to read through the ingredients? Do they look like they were written in a foreign language? Would it be easier to repeat "hippopotamus" three times in a row than sound out one of the ingredients on the stupid label?! If so, then you likely have a bad egg in your hand. Since ingredients are required to be listed in order of volume, if the first five ingredients aren't natural, healthy ingredients, then put the item back and slowly back away from the aisle.

6. BE PREPARED. Stock up on vegan cookbooks. Make grocery and menu lists each week. You are doomed if you plan on wandering around the grocery store and figuring it out on the spot. What you need is a plan. Otherwise those Doritos and shrimp cocktails are going to call your name like a five-dollar hooker. Make a list of all the ingredients you need and what you currently have in your pantry. Rest assured, you will save time, money, and your thighs this way. If you're on a budget, choose ingredients that can be stretched out over a few meals. Trust me, nobody wins in Grocery Roulette.

7. ARM YOURSELF WITH KNOWLEDGE. Know where your nearby natural-food markets are, find the vegan section in your local grocery-store chain (hint: it is usually in the produce refrigerated section), and look into joining a co-op for fresh fruit and vegetable delivery.

8. INVEST IN KITCHEN GADGETS. Become an amateur chef. Get yourself a slow cooker for making hearty delicious meals that simmer while you're at work or school. (For slow cooker recipes, visit crockpot.com and simply veganize the recipes.) Put your money into a food processor for making homemade soups, ice cream, and sauces. Always have a blender for whipping up smoothies and shakes. Consider purchasing a bread maker. It really boils down to how much you cook and what you enjoy cooking, but keep in mind that cooking your own food is a surefire way to achieve healthy vegan status. A bread maker may cost more initially; however, by making your own bread, you have complete control over what goes in it—no chemicals or preservatives. Many bread makers can be used to make pasta as well.

9. WORK A FRUIT OR VEGETABLE INTO EVERY MEAL. This is a great way to get your recommended daily servings throughout the day as well as a low-calorie, healthy meal instead of junk food. You will feel fuller longer, so you won't have to attack the refrigerator like a rabid dog.

10. EAT CONSCIOUSLY, IN EVERY WAY POSSIBLE. Last and certainly not least, be aware of where your food comes from. I cannot stress this

Brands I Trust

After flipping through this book, you'd have to have your head up your ass to not figure out what brands I trust. But just in case this is all too much to take in, here they are spelled out for you:

Eden Organics · Amy's Kitchen · Helen's Kitchen · Road's End · Dr. Oetker · Back to Nature · Food for Life · Bob's Red Mill · Lightlife · Health Is Wealth · Wildwood Organics · Seeds of Change · Arrowhead Mills · WestSoy · Turtle Island Foods · Yves Veggie Cuisine

enough, ladies. Understand what's in your food, what impact it has on the planet and environment, and how it supports your local community. I also suggest doing some research and getting to know the companies that make your favorite products. Learn to support and trust brands that invest in your health instead of lining their own filthy pockets. Act with a conscience.

Transition Foods

For those of you just making the switch to a vegan diet or attempting to eat fewer animal products, I've created a recurring section throughout the book on some of the best transitional foods. These are food products that are so close to the real thing (or better), they make life a tad easier when you're experiencing withdrawals from your usual culinary indulgences. Over the past few years, vegan product manufacturers have gotten real savvy at imitating our favorite conventional foods, so we don't have to deprive our palates. Look for the "Best Transition" product symbol scattered throughout the book.

Decoding the Label
Spotting Animal Ingredients

These days, you need a degree in label reading to decipher what's really lurking in the package. Food manufacturers know what's up—they're not idiots. They're just hoping *you* are. Aside from the hard-to-pronounce words, they use pseudonyms and generic terms that you are familiar with to keep you from asking questions. You name it . . . *caramel coloring, sugar, natural flavoring*. Unfortunately, these broad terms are often just a cover-up for something that used to be an attraction in a petting zoo.

If you're new to shaking your moneymaker on the vegan dance floor, here are a few things to remember when you're skimming over the back of a label.

CHECK FOR CHOLESTEROL. If it's got cholesterol, an animal was involved in some way. In processed foods, animals are the *only* source of cholesterol.

DON'T TRUST THE TERMS "KOSHER" OR "PAREVE." All "kosher" means is that meat and dairy won't be hanging out next to one another in the same dish. "Pareve," on the other hand, just rules out meat or dairy products. But the item may still contain fish, honey, or eggs. Yeah, those jerks are tricky, aren't they?

"NATURAL" DOESN'T EQUAL "VEGAN." Honey is natural. A cow's intestines are natural. But that doesn't mean shit. You don't want to stick either of these in your mouth, if you're going vegan. The only time you should trust this term is when the brand backs it up with hard-core evidence that it's a type of natural you want to eat (or I say you can eat).

DON'T TRUST BROAD TERMS. I already mentioned this one, but be wary of terms like "natural flavor." Chances are that animal parts helped create the flavor. (Many products in this book list "natural flavor" among the ingredients, but don't worry your pretty little head. I've done the research to make sure they're vegan.) Another one is "sugar." White, refined sugar is sometimes produced using animal bone char. Have you ever seen "gum base" or "gelatin" on a label and thrown the item in your cart? Not anymore, kiddo.

BE WARY OF THE "CRUELTY-FREE" LABEL. Now this one is eff'd up. All "cruelty-free" means is that the product wasn't tested on animals, but that doesn't mean there isn't a dead animal in your microwave meal. Plus, this term isn't regulated. Do we have an understanding? Thank you.

DON'T MESS WITH AN INGREDIENT LABELED "NONDAIRY." This term is a result of the efforts of the dairy industry and its lobbying power. Shock-

Honey

Sure, we don't snack on bees or find them in the frozen-food section, but they are still a vegan no-no. Thanks to the demand for a little honey, bees have joined the ranks of the creatures exploited by the factory-farm system, enduring stressful transport and sucky living conditions. They are even starved to death and burned alive by careless beekeepers during unproductive months to limit the dirty work. Does that sound like fun? Yeah, about as much fun as hanging with your grandma on a Saturday night.

Listen, honey, bees pollinate the crops that produce the food you eat. Without them, we'd have a worldwide famine on our hands. Any questions?

ingly, it means diddly-squat. It's really directed at the lactose-intolerant crowd and just means the product is *mostly* free of dairy. You are not all right with "mostly."

If you have an iPhone, download the Vegetarian Scanner application. The app allows you to scan ingredient labels on food products, and it spits out any concerns. Download it on iTunes for $2.99; compatible with iPod touch, iPad, and iPhone iOS 3.1.3 or later.

NICKNAMES FOR ANIMAL INGREDIENTS

ALBUMIN. A protein that comes from eggs or dried blood. Gag me.

CASEIN. A protein that comes from milk and is often hiding in items labeled "nondairy." Not only is this an animal derivative, but studies have shown this icky protein promotes cancer in every stage of development.

COLORING. An additive that may come from insects or bugs. *Ewwww.* If you spot the terms "cochineal" or "carmine," you can be sure you are buying something with ground-up beetles.

GELATIN. A material that comes from animal bones, skin, and connective tissues that are boiled down to the consistency of jelly.

GHEE. An übercommon milk by-product.

HONEY. A sweet fluid that comes from bees. *Obviously.*

LECITHIN. A fat by-product that can come from animal tissues or eggs.

OLEIC ACID. Fat from sheep or cows.

PEPSIN. Heading agent that usually comes from a piggy.

RENNIN/RENNET. An enzyme from a cow's belly.

CALCIUM STEARATE. A mineral often extracted from piggies and cows (the term "calcium" should have tipped you off).

STEARIC ACID. A fat or oil from all types of animals on Old McDonald's farm.

SUGAR. A refined product that is sometimes whitened using bone char.

Dairy Swaps

Cream Cheese

A bagel just isn't the same without a spread of cream cheese. But, as with butter, you might as well eat trash. It contains a shitload of saturated fat and cholesterol and comes from a cow (just in case you slept through elementary school). Regular cream cheese contains 30 percent of your recommended daily value of saturated fat. And that's just the regular. With a flavored variety, the saturated fat is a tad lower, but here's what you're eating for breakfast: milk, milk fat, buttermilk, cheese, salt, and sugar. Sound balanced? Not a chance.

But here's the catch-22: unfortunately, the vegan versions are still on the road to perfection. No big surprise there. Still, some of my favorite alternatives have a creamy texture and mild flavor that work great in a variety of desserts and go well on a bagel with a smidgen of fruit spread.

Swap that

Philadelphia Cream Cheese

for this

Follow Your Heart Cream Cheese

Truth be told, there's no true cream cheese matchup on the market . . . *yet*. But Follow Your Heart Cream Cheese is thick and creamy and spreads as smooth as the real thing. Plus, it has a slightly tangy flavor that makes it my number-one choice for desserts and frostings, hands down (makes a mean cream-cheese frosting for carrot cake). Made with natural, GMO-free, organic goodness (followyourheart.com)!

Tofutti Better Than Cream Cheese

If you like a firmer cream cheese rather than the whipped kind, Tofutti Better Than Cream Cheese is your *wo*man. It's not the healthiest choice on the planet, since it contains sugar and some fatty ingredients, but, like traditional cream cheese, it's fine in moderation, and it's nice to have some different flavors, so you don't get bored. Available in Nonhydrogenated Plain, French Onion, Herbs and Chive, and Garlic and Herb (tofutti.com).

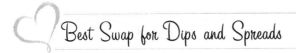

Best Swap for Dips and Spreads

*Galaxy Foods Vegan Cream Cheese

An amazing gluten-free spread with no GMOs or hydrogenated oils. The Chive and Garlic flavor is paradigm for spinach and artichoke dips. Available in Classic Plain or Chive and Garlic (galaxyfoods.com).

Cheese

When making the vegan transition, cheese is always the toughest to let go of. And there's a fabulous reason for that. I'd rather lick a seat on a crowded public bus than eat the stuff that passed as "cheese alternatives" a few years ago. Plus, it wouldn't melt if you left it in a 100-degree car for thirty minutes with the windows rolled up. Okay, I'm a bit of a drama queen, but my, oh my, have things changed. Thanks to the brands below, I can still make nachos, veggie burgers, pizza, quiche—you name it—without gagging. And you college girls can still stuff your face with mac 'n' cheese after you've had a few too many vodka cocktails at the bar. I consider that a blessing. Mark my words, you will too.

An asterisk (*) means the product is gluten-free.

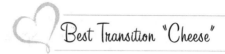

Swap that ∿∿

Shredded cheese

for this

Daiya Cheese

Daiya is the bee's knees. The plant-based, soy-free cheese that I so dare to call an "alternative" comes in shredded cheddar and Italian blends in a bag; it melts like a champ, but without the artificial ingredients, preservatives, or cholesterol. The cheddar has a nice rich and sharp flavor that gives burritos and quesadillas a punch. Tofurky and Daiya have even teamed up for a line of frozen vegan pizzas (I'll get to those). Over-the-moon delicious (daiyafoods.com).

Swap that ∿∿

Block cheese

for this

Follow Your Heart Cheese

My second favorite next to Daiya, this rich, cheddary vegan cheese comes in blocks, but shreds nicely too. Made from soybeans and expeller-pressed canola oil, Follow Your Heart's cheese requires higher temperatures to melt, but hey, it still melts. Don't get too picky. Available in Cheddar, Mozzarella, Monterey Jack, and Nacho (followyourheart.com).

Best Appetizer Cheese

Dr. Cow Aged Vegan Cheese

Your mom always told you that you were "different" from the rest. Well, sweetheart, meet your match. This line of aged gluten-free cheese blocks is made with cashew nuts, Brazil nuts, and macadamia nuts; some varieties have kale, dulse, and hemp seeds thrown in. The sharp flavor is tough to describe, but slice it up next to some fancy crackers or toasted French bread, and I guarantee your guests won't give a rat's ass what's in it. Each block is 100 percent organic, with no additives or artificial ingredients, and loaded with vitamins, minerals, and essential fatty acids. Available in Aged Cashew Nut, Aged Cashew and Crystal Algae, Aged Cashew and Brazil Nut, Aged Cashew and Dulse, Aged Cashew and Hemp Seeds, Aged Cashew and Kale, Aged Macadamia Nut, and Aged Macadamia and Hemp (dr-cow.com).

Swap that

for this

Cheezly, Mature Cheddar Style

With a distinct, sharp cheese flavor, Cheezly makes a kick-ass grilled cheese sandwich. It comes in block form or slices and doesn't melt quite like Daiya, but, let's face it, few do. Also available in Edam Style, Garlic and Herb Flavor, Gouda Style, Nacho Style, Mozzarella Style, and Added Bacon Style Pieces (not real bacon, dingo; redwoodfoods.es).

▸ *Sharpest cheddar flavor on the vegan shelf!*

*Galaxy Foods Vegan Rice Cheese Slices

Veggie cheese slices made with organic ingredients. Free of soy and gluten. Available in Cheddar and American (galaxyfoods.com).

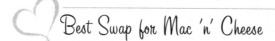 Best Swap for Mac 'n' Cheese

Teese Cheese

This one is great for kids, especially those with food allergies (it's made in a facility with no egg, dairy, peanut, tree nut, or sesame in the vicinity). The texture is smooth with a mild, slightly buttery flavor that the whole family will love—vegan or not. Break it up into smaller pieces in a pan with noodles to achieve a more creamy consistency, and it makes a supreme mac 'n' cheese. Teese Cheese is made from non-GMO soybeans and is also low in fat. Available in Mozzarella, Cheddar, Nacho Sauce, and Creamy Cheddar Sauce (teesecheese.com).

Swap that

Cheese flakes and sprinkles

for this

*Eat in the Raw Parma Vegan Parmesan

Sprinkle this vegan parmesan powder on pasta, pizza, vegetables, and popcorn. It's gluten-free and a healthy source of omega-3s and vitamin B-12. Available in Chipotle Cayenne and Original (eatintheraw.com).

Dairy Free Parmazano Grated
Hard Cheese Replacer

This comes in a nifty shaker bottle (like the Eat in the Raw) with a rich, cheesy flavor. No GMOs or hydrogenated oils (store.vegan essentials.com).

Food Dyes

Need another reason to avoid Kraft? Most store-bought cheeses contain artificial food dyes. For kids, exposure to food dyes has been linked to hyperactivity (ADHD), cancer, and severe food allergies. The food giant has been getting a lot of heat for using artificial food dyes in its U.S.-marketed products, yet it reformulates them for the European market due to consumer pressure. Apparently, we're chopped liver over here in the States.

Swap that

Cheese mixes

for this

*Road's End Organics Cheddar "Chreese" Sauce Mixes

No, I didn't spell "cheese" wrong. Road's End did. *Duh.* These versatile cheese mixes come in envelopes for individual servings or family-size one-pound bags, depending on how many mouths you're feeding. I find them particularly great for making pizza and lasagna or melting on chips, crackers, and vegetables. Another plus? They can be stored in the refrigerator for ten to fourteen days after preparing. Available in Cheddar Chreese (both original and gluten-free), Mozzarella Chreese, and Alfredo Style (edwardandsons.com).

Yogurt

Yogurt is one of the best snacks a woman can nosh on. It contains active cultures that stop all that bad bacteria from camping out in your body, and it's packed with healthy nutrients. It can also help fight yeast and urinary tract infections when you have some problems "down under." But it doesn't take a rocket scientist to figure out that it's made from fermented milk. Yeah, not vegan, kiddo. Many of the vegan yogurts in the grocery store today contain many of the same benefits, but without the udder juice.

Swap that ↝↝↝↝↝

Yoplait

↜↜↜↜↜ for this

*So Delicious Coconut Milk Yogurt

Even your hubby will dump the Yoplait after trying this coconut yogurt. It totally looks like regular yogurt, with a thick and creamy consistency—not all watery and thin like some imitation yogurts. (My son loves it!) Choose from GMO-free, soy-based or soy-free yogurts and smoothies that are so creamy and flavorful. Available in a variety of flavors including Chocolate, Strawberry-Banana, Blueberry, Passionate Mango, Vanilla, Raspberry, and Pina Colada (turtlemountain.com).

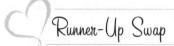

Runner-Up Swap

*Whole Soy & Co. Yogurt

Your choices are not limited with this soy yogurt made with natural colors, evaporated cane sugar, and organic, non-GMO soybeans grown on a farm in northwestern Texas. You still get your live cultures and added calcium. Available in plain and unsweetened or eleven delicious fruity flavors including Cherry, Key Lime, and Apricot Mango (wholesoyco.com).

KIM'S PICK: When I was pregnant, I used to waddle out of Whole Foods with cases of the Vanilla yogurt; it was so good sprinkled with some pumpkin seeds for a snack.

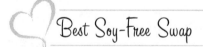

Best Soy-Free Swap

*Ricera Rice Yogurt

For those who hate or are allergic to soy, each of Ricera's organic yogurts delivers one and a half servings of whole-grain rice with active cultures and no GMOs. It's thinner in consistency and a bit on the watery side, but it still tastes scrumptious. Available in Strawberry, Blueberry, Peach, and Vanilla (ricerafoods.com).

Silk Live! Soy Yogurt

This soy-based yogurt line is pumped with beneficial probiotics and comes in a handful of creamy varieties, including Blueberry, Black Cherry, Key Lime, Peach, Raspberry, Strawberry, Banana-Strawberry, Vanilla, and Plain (silksoymilk.com).

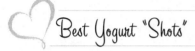

Best Yogurt "Shots"

GoodBelly

Hold it right there—in the spirit of transparency, this isn't yogurt. It's so much better. This is a certified organic juice with live and active probiotic cultures to balance the good and bad bacteria. For you bar-flies, it comes in "shot form." Just rip back the lid and chug-a-lug, baby. Available in cool flavors such as Pomegranate Blackberry, Cranberry Watermelon, Mango, Blueberry Acai, Lemon Ginger, Vanilla Chamomile, and Strawberry. GoodBelly ToGo Powder is gluten-free and only available online (goodbelly.com).

Milk

Milk doesn't do anybody's body good. It comes with a fair share of cholesterol and saturated fat, not to mention it contains casein. Let me tell you about casein. It's a protein found in 87 percent of cow's milk that has been shown to promote cancer in all stages of development. Yeah, I'll pass. I plan on sticking around and annoying the hell out of carnivores for the

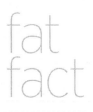

Leave it to the dairy industry to trick chicks into believing that milk prevents osteoporosis. Drinking milk doesn't prevent bone loss, bitches. In fact, bone loss is accelerated by ingesting too much protein, too much of this thing with the nickname "liquid meat." That's what a huge marketing budget and a great advertising agency will do for you.

next sixty years. No matter your preferences, milk alternatives now come in a number of varieties. Take your pick.

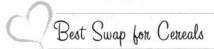

Best Swap for Cereals

Soy Milk

The most common dairy substitute available, soy milk is a great source of essential amino acids, potassium, and iron. Soy milk is also chock-full of bioactive components, which help maintain healthy bones and relieve menopausal symptoms and hot flashes.

Pacific Natural Foods Soymilk

Available in Select Plain, Select Vanilla, and Unsweetened Original (pacificfoods.com).

Silk Soymilk

Available in GMO-free, certified organic varieties, including Organic Vanilla, Organic Original, and Organic Unsweetened. If you want something on the light side, stick with Silk Light, sweetened with stevia for no added calories. Simply Silk flavors include Original, Chocolate, Strawberry, Vanilla, and Very Vanilla (silksoymilk.com).

Soy Dream

Available in nonrefrigerated and refrigerated versions such as Classic Vanilla, Enriched Chocolate, Enriched Original, and Enriched Vanilla (tastethedream.com).

"Milk" Tips

If soy ain't your thang, almond milk is another great milk alternative for cereals or dunking cookies. The best "milks" for making desserts or hot chocolate are vanilla or sweetened almond milk, soy milk, and rice milk. Hemp and hazelnut milks are ideal for baking nut breads, since they have a sweet, nutty taste.

Almond Milk

Most people agree almond milk tastes the closest to cow's milk. It has a rich and creamy taste like milk but is lower in calories and fat. Almond milk is also high in antioxidants and vitamin D, but it's the balance of protein, monounsaturated "good" fats, and fiber in almonds that may help you lose weight.

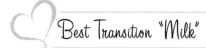 Best Transition "Milk"

Blue Diamond Almond Breeze

My personal favorite (and my son's), because it's not too thick and not too watery. Blue Diamond has a rich, creamy texture, and it goes down *sooo* smooth. Available in Original, Original Unsweetened, Chocolate, Chocolate Unsweetened, Vanilla, and Vanilla Unsweetened (blue diamond.com).

Silk Pure Almond

Available in Original, Vanilla, Dark Chocolate, and Unsweetened (silkpurealmond.com).

Almond Dream

An enriched almond milk available in Original and Original Unsweetened (both fortified with calcium and vitamins B-12 and D), Unsweetened Vanilla, and Vanilla (tastethedream.com).

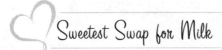 Sweetest Swap for Milk

Rice Milk

Derived from brown rice, rice milk is naturally sweeter with a thinner texture than soy or almond milk. Commercial brands are often fortified with calcium, iron, and vitamins A, D, and B.

Rice Dream

Made by the same company that produces Soy Dream, Rice Dream comes in both nonrefrigerated and refrigerated versions, including Carob, Enriched Chocolate, Enriched Original, Enriched Vanilla, Heartwise Original, Heartwise Vanilla, Horchata (aye, aye, aye!), Original, and Supreme Chocolate Chai (tastethedream.com).

Pacific Natural Foods Rice Milk

With no added sugar, only the sweetness that comes from the brown rice, Pacific Rice Milk is available in All Natural Rice Plain and All Natural Rice Vanilla (pacificfoods.com).

Hemp Milk

Laugh it up, stoners. You are more than welcome to have a glass at 4:20 P.M., but hemp milk is made from the seeds of the hemp plant. No THC included. It has a creamy nutty flavor, making it a prime candidate for baking, and is high in essential amino acids, potassium, and folic acid.

Pacific Natural Foods Hemp Milk

Available in Original, Hemp Vanilla, and Hemp Chocolate (pacific foods.com).

Hemp Dream

Hemp Dream is high in omega-3s and -6s and comes in cool psyche-delic packaging. Available in Original and Vanilla (tastethedream.com).

Hazelnut Milk

Low in fat with no saturated fat or cholesterol, Hazelnut isn't the most popular milk alternative on the market, but it's a nice choice for baking.

Pacific Natural Foods Hazelnut Milk

Available in All Natural Hazelnut Original, All Natural Hazelnut Chocolate (also in single serve; pacificfoods.com).

Drinks on the Go

Whether it's a road trip or you're just late for work, to-go drink boxes are great for kids and traveling. Look for these at your local grocer or natural-foods retailer or online at amazon.com:

ZenSoy Soy on the Go Soymilk, available in Vanilla and Chocolate.

Rice Dream Rice Drink, 8-ounce boxes, available in Enriched Original, Enriched Vanilla, and Enriched Chocolate.

Pacific Natural Foods drinks, 8-ounce boxes, available in Organic Almond and Lowfat Chocolate.

Sour Cream

Besides the mere fact that it contains dairy, sour cream gets 90 percent of its calories from fat. Considering that 2 tablespoons only offer an average of 52 calories, that's not so bad. But when you find that at least half of that fat is saturated, bad is exactly what it is. Saturated fat is the stuff that screws up your health and prompts strangers at the airport to ask if you're having a boy or a girl. Don't look at them like they're assholes—you're the one dumping it all over your enchiladas. Try one of these vegan alternatives, which deliver a quarter of the saturated fat and are made with all-natural, animal-friendly ingredients.

Swap that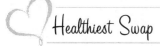

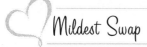 for this

*Follow Your Heart Sour Cream Alternative

Follow Your Heart's sour cream is full-bodied and creamy, but lacks the sourness of traditional sour cream. I've never been a fan of the sour bite, so I actually prefer it. The line is derived from non-GMO soybeans and sweetened with organic agave syrup (followyourheart.com).

Mildest Swap

Tofutti Sour Supreme

Tofutti's dairy-free sour cream has a really mild flavor and no weird taste. It gets its texture and zesty flavor from soybeans and tofu (tofutti.com).

Healthiest Swap

*Wayfare Foods We Can't Say It's Sour Cream

This sour cream alternative tastes the most natural, and it's about as healthy as you're going to get. No gluten, GMOs, hydrogenated oils, or crazy colors and flavors (wayfarefoods.com).

Egg and Meat Swaps

Hollah! Vegan Staple

Eggs

They may not look or feel like meat, but those things that pop out of a chicken's ass are not exempt from being produced under cruel conditions. Hens live in batteries of wire cages their entire lives. Usually packed twelve birds to a cage, they are never able to spread their wings (tough to do in a cage roughly 18 to 20 inches wide).

Do me a favor, and don't buy into the "cage-free" mumbo jumbo either. There is no legal definition of the term, which often means that hens are packed side by side in massive sheds or mud-filled lots with only a teeny-weeny opening to the outdoors. They can still be debeaked, a very painful process, and pumped with hormones, so they grow bigger and bigger. Plus, here's a little secret: there are often more stress-related hormones in the eggs of cage-free chickens than in those from battery hens, because the flock is too big for the chickens to establish a pecking order. Did you order some pain and suffering with your omelet? Didn't think so. Luckily, you're not devoid of a good tofu scramble, thanks to egg replacers.

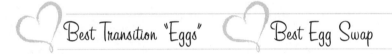

*Ener-G Egg Replacer

This is my first choice when it comes to egg replacers (in reality, however, there are few options). Make sure to mix the powder and water well, so you aren't left with a chalky aftertaste (ener-g.com).

Bob's Red Mill Egg Replacer

Made from soy and wheat, this eggless powder has a nice texture and is great for baked goods like cakes, pancakes, waffles, and muffins (bobsredmill.com).

*Orgran Natural Egg Replacer

A no-egg powder that makes a mean replacement for eggs in baking, especially for fillings and custards. Contains no gluten or wheat—made

An asterisk (*) means the product is gluten-free.

Egg Alternatives

If egg replacers freak you out, try using some of these unconventional ingredients in place of eggs:

For Desserts or Baked Goods

1 egg = 1 banana

1 egg = ½ cup applesauce

1 egg = 1 cup milk substitute plus 1 teaspoon apple cider vinegar

2 or 3 eggs = 1 tablespoon mild-flavored vinegar combined with nondairy milk (soymilk is best) to curdle and produce 1 cup; this works best in a recipe that also calls for baking soda

For Breakfast or Everyday Dishes

1 egg = ½ cup silken tofu

1 egg = 2 tablespoons potato starch

1 egg = ½ cup mashed potatoes

1 egg = 2 tablespoons water, 1 tablespoon olive oil, and 2 teaspoons baking soda

When using tofu, be sure to puree it first so you don't have chunks in the final dish. Hey, it should look pretty too.

in an Aussie facility that makes sure there is no cross-contamination (orgran.com).

PaneRiso Foods Egg Replacer

This boxed egg replacer mix equals 100 eggs (canbrands.ca).

— THE SKINNY —

Tofu for Tat

Firm. Extra firm. Soft. Silken. Sounds dirty, but what the hell does it all mean? Here are the best tofu pairings for all styles of cooking:

Firm/Extra Firm: Best for stir-fries, salads, and pasta salads, and cut in cubes for snacking; also delish when fried (makes the best fried "egg" sandwiches).

Medium: Best for tofu scrambles, burritos, tacos, chili, and lasagna.

Soft/Silken: Best for smoothies, dips, soups, and as an egg replacer when baking.

Hollah! Vegan Staple

Tofu

Tofu gives a lot of people the heebie-jeebies. Not just because it looks like chalk, but because they don't know what the hell to do with it. When I first made the crossover, I would just stare at it in my fridge like it was a child in a bar. It just didn't make sense. But all you have to do is give it a good soak in a marinade and then stir-fry, grill, or bake it, and you'll start to look at it as you would a hot bartender in a bar: ready for some action.

Tofu is a great source of protein for vegans, plus it is high in tryptophan, iron, omega-3 fatty acids, and calcium. It adds some substance to a meal without the cholesterol or extra serving of sugar and artificial sugars. Quit being a pussy and just try to cook with it; you'll find it's almost foolproof if you follow just a few directions.

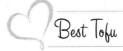 Best Tofu

Nasoya Sprouted Tofu

The tofu maker with arguably the most cred, Nasoya produces tofu made from organic sprouted soybeans with no preservatives. Choose from Organic Sprouted Tofu Super Firm, Extra Firm, Firm, Soft, Silken, Lite Firm, Cubes, and Lite Silken. Nasoya also makes tofu fortified with vitamins in firm and extra firm (nasoya.com).

Wildwood Organics SprouTofu

Made with sprouted soybeans, SprouTofu comes in Silken, Super Firm, and Extra Firm in a handful of different flavors such as Plain, Baked, Golden, and Smoked. With the ready-mades, you don't even have to go through the trouble of marinating. Choose from Aloha Baked, Royal Thai Baked, Golden Pineapple Teriyaki, Garlic Teriyaki Smoked, and Hickory BBQ Smoked (pulmuonewildwood.com).

House Foods Tofu

House Foods carries seasoned tofu, including Tofu Steak Grilled and Tofu Steak Cajun, but its specialty is options. You can't go wrong with its wide variety of textures, sizes, and degrees of firmness. Choose from Premium Tofu Soft, Medium, Firm, Extra Soft, Extra Firm and Organic Tofu Soft, Medium, and Firm (house-foods.com).

Ground Beef

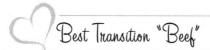 Best Transition "Beef"

Yves Meatless Ground Round Original

These meatless crumbles have the consistency, texture, and flavor of ground beef, but with none of the saturated fat, cholesterol, or preservatives. They're precooked and perfect for stir-fries, tacos, quesadillas, sloppy joes, and salads (yvesveggie.com).

When substituting a vegan meat for real meat, as a general rule use the same amount. In laywoman's terms, if a recipe calls for 4 ounces of ground beef, use 4 ounces of fake beef.

Lifelight Smart Ground Original

Make it Taco Tuesday every night. These veggie crumbles make some bomb-ass tacos, but they're also wildly divine in lettuce wraps. Also available in Mexican and Tex Mex (lightlife.com).

*Dixie Diner Beef (Not!) Ground

Imitation beef that is gluten-free and low in sodium, fat, and sugar. By the looks of it, it kind of resembles dog food, so don't judge this book by its cover. Also available in Beef (Not!) Strips and Beef (Not!) Chunks (dixiediner.com).

⫸ *Not a beef eater? Go for the "turkey" flavor! Like the beef, the Turkey (Not!) Ground comes in crumbles that are great for salads, stir-fries, breakfast scrambles, and casseroles. Low in sodium and gluten-free.*

Canned Beef

Cedar Lake Meatless Beef Strips

Beef in a can? You betcha. These tender strips make for the perfect fajitas (cedarlakefoods.com).

Worthington Choplets

Precooked, canned cutlets in a vegetable broth. These taste best when you bread them with spices and serve on a whole-grain bun (worthingtonfoods.com).

Seitan

Let's be real: beef is boring. You can marinate, soak it, and season it like crazy, and you still taste a dead cow. But with seitan and tempeh you call the shots. You can master any flavor you want with the right preparation methods and seasonings. And there's a bonus: you don't fill up on saturated fat and cholesterol. Um, awesome.

Seitan is made from gluten, it's low fat, and it scores high in the protein department. In fact, it has about the same amount of protein as beef and twice as much as tofu. For those making the vegan transition or just trying to cut their intake of animal-based products, it's firm and texturized to feel like meat in your mouth. Because that's what it's all about, isn't it?

White Wave Chicken-Style Wheat Meat

A fake meat made of wheat gluten, pea starch, and garbanzo bean flour. Add it to stir-fries in place of chicken (foodservicedirect.com).

Everyday Uses for Seitan

Don't just let it sit there and look pretty. Work seitan into dishes such as soups, stews, Chinese stir-fries, casseroles, and BBQ sandwiches. By itself, it tastes a little bland. But when you marinate it, it takes on any disguise you like.

WestSoy Chicken-Style Seitan Seasoned Wheat Protein

Another great chicken replacement for stir-fries and juicy fajitas (foodservicedirect.com).

WestSoy Traditional Seasoned Seitan

These chicken-style chunks are pretty high in protein (18 grams per serving) and precooked, so little prep is required (foodservicedirect .com).

Upton's Naturals Seitan

A GMO-free meat alternative made of vital wheat gluten, soy sauce, spices, and whole-wheat flour. Try the Traditional Style, Chorizo-Style (dee-lish for breakfast burritos and tacos), Ground Beef–Style (excel-

Everyday Uses for Tempeh

Tempeh is a cinch to cook with. It's made from whole soybeans and fermented into a cake patty. I love to marinate it in coconut milk or oil, peanut sauce, or Tamari sauce and gently blacken it on the grill or in a pan. Add it to casseroles, chili, and Mexican dishes or slice it up into thin strips for some tasty bacon. (I have some specific tempeh recommendations in the Bacon section.)

lent in sloppy joes, tacos, and meatloaf), and Italian Sausage–Style (mmm . . . pizza topping; uptonsnaturals.com).

Tempeh

There's a reason this stuff has been around for thousands of years. It's healthy. It's better naked than seitan. (It's got a chewy texture like beef jerky, but a mild, nutty flavor.) And it has some cool effects on your body. Tempeh isn't just one of those crunchy, hippie foods that only tree huggers and vegans like. Gassy, bloated people like it too. Yeah, I said it—the oligosaccharides in beans, legumes, and soy are tough for some people to digest. But the fermentation process that tempeh goes through greatly reduces the number of oligosaccharides, so it "goes down" easier. There are also enzymes in tempeh that help increase the absorption of minerals.

WestSoy Tempeh Five Grain

Tempeh made with organic soy beans and grains. Read: no GMOs. Great for stir-fries. Also available in Original (amazon.com).

Lightlife Organic Tempeh

With more than thirty years' experience making tempeh, Lightlife shines, with six different gourmet varieties. Each one has a nutritious yet bold flavor that spices up any meal. Available in Flax, Garden Veggie, Soy, Smoky Strips, Three Grain, and Wild Rice (lightlife.com).

Turtle Island Foods Marinated Tempeh

Regular tempeh is so old-school. So Tofurky stepped in and sliced organic soy tempeh into thin strips and marinated it in four flavors for more distinguished tastes. Available in Coconut Curry, Sesame Garlic, Lemon Pepper, and Smoky Apple Bacon (tofurky.com).

Although fake beef is a kick-ass transition food when you're removing the real stuff from your diet, it's not the only substitution. If a recipe calls for beef, cutlets, or sirloin, swap out for portobello mushrooms instead. On that note, if you never tried a portobello cheesesteak, you are missing out, sister.

Beef Jerky

I'm not afraid to admit that I mourn the loss of some of America's best yet worst culinary creations. One in particular: beef jerky. Excuse my language, but jerky is effing divine. A road trip was not a white-trash road trip without a few sticks in my lap and one shredded between my teeth (and Pat Benatar on full blast). But when it really hit me that I was sucking on dehydrated meat that is cured with sodium chloride and loaded with preservatives, I cut all ties. A travesty? You don't know the half of it. But I couldn't stay away for long. Beef jerky is stuck on me, and I'm stuck on it. So rather than avoid it like a heart attack, I decided to find healthier brands that wouldn't harden my arteries. A match made in jerky heaven.

Swap that

Jack Links Beef Jerky

for this

Tasty Eats Soy Jerky

Me. My husband. My son. We're all terribly addicted to this soy jerky, and rightfully so. It contains no cholesterol, preservatives, MSG, or GMOs, and it's low in fat. Available in Original, Peppered, Teriyaki, Cajun Chick'n, and Hot N' Spicy (tastyeats.com).

KIM'S PICK: Teriyaki—a succulent combo of sweet and rugged.

Swap that ⟲⟲⟲

⟲⟲⟲ for this

Primal Spirit Primal Strips

These single-serve meatless jerky strips are long and thin just like the junk we used to chew on at Little League, but without the preservatives or artificial colors. They have a spicy, hickory flavor, and even the texture comes off as meaty. If you fall into the outdoorsy category, just throw them in your backpack for some protein post–mountain climb, swim, or whatever crazy hobby that you get off on. Available in Thai Peanut (seitan), Mesquite Lime (seitan), Teriyaki (seitan), Hot and Spicy (shiitake mushrooms), Hickory Smoked (soy), and Texas BBQ (soy; primalspiritfoods.com).

Tofurky Jurky

Made in a real smokehouse, Tofurky jerky is marinated in a GMO-free soy sauce, garlic, lemon juice, and organic evaporated cane juice, before it is slowly smoked to awesomeness. Available in Original and Peppered (tofurky.com).

Vegan Dream Vegetarian Jerky

This one isn't so easy to find, but I threw it in here for you crazies who like a challenge. Available in Original Hickory Pepper, Cowgirl, Hot Chili Pepper, and Teriyaki (the last one has psyllium husk as an ingredient, which adds a little fiber to the jerky; vegandream.com).

Bacon

Lightlife Organic Smoky Tempeh Strips, Fakin' Bacon

Certified organic tempeh with a smoky flavor. It doesn't matter how you eat it or what you eat it with—it's that good (lightlife.com).

Best Transition "Bacon"

Swap that ∞∞∞

Bacon strips

∞∞∞ *for this*

Lightlife Smart Bacon Bacon-Style Strips

These strips look like turkey bacon. They taste like turkey bacon. But you guessed it . . . they're not turkey bacon. We're talking crispy, non-greasy veggie bacon without the saturated fat or cholesterol. Smart Bacon, 1; real bacon, 0 (lightlife.com).

Swap that

for this

Yves Meatless Canadian Bacon

Smoky Canadian bacon with a blend of bold spices that will turn any Eggs Benedict upside down (yvesveggie.com).

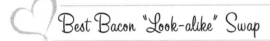

Best Bacon "Look-alike" Swap

May Wah Vegan Bacon Strips

Breaking the mold, May Wah's "bacon" is made of red yeast, mushrooms, and seaweed, giving it an Asian twist (vegieworld.com).

Best Flavor Swap

Turtle Island Foods Smoky Maple Bacon Marinated Tempeh

Flavored bacon that will wake up any ole BLT. It's got the same chewy texture as bacon, but with a hint of sweetness thanks to the maple marinade. Pair it with a stack of pancakes, sweet cheeks (tofurky.com).

Frontier Bac'Uns Organic Vegan Bacon Bits

Organic, crumbled soy bacon perfect for salads, tofu scrambles, and soups (frontiercoop.com).

Sausage

Save a pig, eat a fake one. That's my motto. And because of the brave folks below who dared to go where not many food manufacturers have dared to go, I can say it with attitude.

Tofurky Italian Sausages

Sweet Italian sausages blended with sun-dried tomatoes and basil (tofurky.com).

Match Vegan Sausages

Match makes gourmet plant-based meats like nobody else. Expect a similar taste and consistency minus the hormones and antibiotics that come with products from the modern-day food system. The Italian Vegan Sausage is a perfect addition to pasta dishes, while the Breakfast Sausage patties make an awesome side (matchmeats.com).

Swap that ⦿⦿⦿⦿

Sausage

⦿⦿⦿⦿ *for this*

Lightlife Gimme Lean Sausage

Ground "sausage" that can be sautéed chunky-style for things like tacos and casseroles or crafted into any form or shape such as burger patties—with zero fat. Yes, a big fat 0. My son has been eating this for years, and he just can't get enough. Available in Ground Sausage Style and Ground Beef Style (lightlife.com).

Swap that ⦿⦿⦿⦿

Chorizo

⦿⦿⦿⦿ *for this*

El Burrito Soyrizo

Made with 100 percent soybeans, this Mexican-style sausage alternative is disturbingly close to authentic chorizo. OMG. It's a little soft and squishy, but when pan-fried, it hardens up for a meaty texture. Soyrizo also has a nice little kick, which makes it taste like it was made for paella dishes (elburrito.com).

Swap that 〜〜〜

Sausage links

〜〜〜 *for this*

Lightlife Smart Links Breakfast Sausage Style

Man, does Lightlife have a knack for imitating meat, or does Lightlife have a knack for imitating meat?! Its signature meatless sausage links are a dead ringer for traditional sausage. Only 3 grams of fat per serving (lightlife.com).

Best Transition "Sausage Dogs"

Swap that 〜〜〜

Gourmet sausage

〜〜〜 *for this*

Field Roast Grain Meat Sausages

If you want to convince any meat eater that vegans don't make many sacrifices, grill up one of these gourmet sausage alternatives. It's juicy yet firm, adventurous yet sophisticated, and packs tons of flavor from roasted vegetables, fruits, and seeds. Available in Italian, Mexican Chipotle, and Smoked Apple Sage (fieldroast.com).

KIM'S PICKS: I love the spiciness of the Mexican Chipotle, and the Smoked Apple Sage is the perfect touch for a Sunday brunch.

Tofurky Kielbasa

A meatless imitation of the Polish staple seasoned with onion and garlic (tofurky.com).

Tofurky Breakfast Links

Soy links with bold, peppery flavors. Great in a morning scramble (tofurky.com).

Hot Dogs

Tofu Franks *and* Vege-Dogs

Meatless dogs with light seasoning (cedarlakefoods.com).

SoyBoy Vegetarian Franks

A healthy hot dog? Believe it, sister. SoyBoy's meatless franks contain no preservatives, little fat and sodium, and nothin' artificial (soy boy.com).

Swap that ∿∿∿

Beef hot dogs

∿∿∿ for this

Lightlife Smart Dogs

Take yourself out to the ball game with these veggie protein links. They have a softer texture than some of the other protein dogs, but the flavor is right on. Think nice and meaty with a smoky flavor. They also come in jumbo, if you like 'em big (lightlife.com).

Lightlife Original Tofu Pups

Tofu dogs rich in protein and low in fat (lightlife.com).

Canned Worthington Loma Linda Big Franks

Who doesn't love a can of weenies? These have a smoky flavor like Polish sausage and are excellent on the grill (worthingtonfoods.com).

Cedar Lake Meatless Tofu Links

Fat-free canned tofu dogs made from wheat, soy isolate, and tofu (cedarlakefoods.com).

Swap that ∽∽∽∽

Turkey dogs

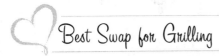 for this

Tofurky Franks

Thick, firm, and meaty franks with a hint of turkey flavor that will shake up any carnivore (tofurky.com).

Yves Veggie Brats

I thought the day would never come. And, damn, am I glad I was wrong. Yves's newest miracle, meatless brats, rack up less than 100 calories, and they're grill-ready. Available in Classic and Zesty Italian (yvesveggie.com).

Best Swap for Grilling

Yves Meatless Hot Dog

Fire up the grill, bitches. These have a texture firm enough to withstand the pressures of the grill, and the barbecue really enhances the natural hickory flavor and spice blend. They're also low in calories and fat, if you're counting. Also available in Jumbo, which is 60 percent bigger (yvesveggie.com)!

Burgers

Swap that

Meat burger patties

for this

Boca Original Vegan Meatless Burgers

Boca has the meatiest and smokiest flavor of the bunch. I'll admit, they may be a little on the dry side, but they're delicious jazzed up with some tomatoes, pickles, and ketchup (bocaburger.com).

Best Burger for a Meat Eaters' Cookout

MorningStar Farms Grillers Vegan Veggie Burgers

These might just be my favorite for entertaining nonvegan guests during a good ole-fashioned cookout. They're meaty, smoky, and grill-tastic. Just top with your favorite condiments, and you've got a killer burger with 84 percent less fat than a dead animal (morningstar farms.com).

Swap that ͡°͡°͡°͡°

͡°͡°͡°͡° *for this*

Boca Spicy Chik'N Patties

These breaded meatless chicken patties are moist on the inside with a spicy, crispy goodness on the outside (bocaburger.com).

Chicken Nuggets

Swap that ͡°͡°͡°͡°

Chicken nuggets

͡°͡°͡°͡° *for this*

Health Is Wealth Chicken-Free Nuggets

Want to make the kids feel like they're eating fast food? Bingo, mama! These 100 percent vegetable nuggets will appeal to even the pickiest of nugget lovers. They have an authentic juicy chicken flavor wrapped in a crispy breading made with stone-ground whole wheat (healthiswealthfoods.com).

Mon Cuisine Vegan Chicken Nuggets

Soy-based nuggets breaded and fried with expeller-pressed canola oil. No bogus colors, flavors, or preservatives, just the good stuff. Also available in Breaded Chicken Style Cutlets (alleprocessing.com/alle).

May Wah Vegan Chicken Nuggets

These remind me of McDonald's chicken nuggets, which I loved as a kid. But then I found one in my Happy Meal that was mysteriously shaped like a real baby chicken, and that was all she wrote (or ate). These come without the guilt (vegieworld.com).

Chicken Strips

MorningStar Farms Meal Starters Chik'n Strips

Grilled veggie strips that are lightly seasoned with herbs and spices. Only 140 calories in twelve strips (morningstarfarms.com).

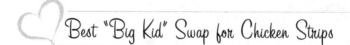

Best "Big Kid" Swap for Chicken Strips

Gardein Chipotle Lime Crispy Fingers

Probably the closest thing I have tasted to real chicken strips à la theme-park style. They have a slightly zesty chipotle kick that might be too much for the kiddies, but there is no doubt that these finger foods will impress your meat-eating friends. Plus, they are ready in ten minutes—that's my kind of quickie (gardein.com).

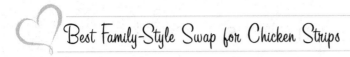

Best Family-Style Swap for Chicken Strips

Lifelight Smart Strips Chick'n Style Strips

Thin, sleek, moist strips of "chicken" that are great in stir-fries, salads, and veggie wraps. They're also great à la carte with your favorite sauce for dipping. But if dip and gorge is more your style, you might like the Smart Tenders in Savory Chick'n and Lemon Pepper. (Also available in *Steak Style Strips*! A dead ringer for the veggie "chicken" strips, but in a juicy, steak flavor; lightlife.com).

Harvest Direct Soy Chicken

Shake up your routine with this GMO-free soy "chicken" in Chunk Style, Strip Style, and Breast Style (dixiediner.com).

*Butler Soy Curls

Fake chicken with style. These curls look like Fritos, but have the texture of real chicken. One hundred percent natural ingredients and gluten-free (butlerfoods.com).

fat
fact

In America, 59 percent of vegetarians are chicks, and 41 percent are dudes.

Wings, Drumsticks, and Ribs

Swap that ∿∿∿

Buffalo wings

∿∿∿ *for this*

Gardein Meat Free Wings

Whether it's the Classic Style Buffalo Wings or Sweet and Tangy Barbecue Wings, these boneless (duh!) wings nail the meat category. They are loaded with good ingredients, including soy, wheat gluten, and ancient grains such as kamut, amaranth, millet, and quinoa. And the sauce really seals the deal—the Classic Style is spicier, and the Sweet and Tangy is milder, with a blend of Dijon mustard, molasses, chili powder, garlic, and hickory smoke. All you need is a cold beer, and you're set (gardein.com).

♡ *Runner-Up Swap*

Health Is Wealth Chicken-Free Buffalo Wings

In a close second, these chickenless buffalo wings have a saucy, chewy texture. Oh, and they're also low-fat and GMO-free, with purely natural ingredients (healthiswealthfoods.com).

VegeCyber Vegan Drum Sticks

Sorry, KFC. These fried chicken drumsticks are a basic blend of soy, wheat protein, flour, bamboo shoot, sugar cane, and vegetable seasoning (vegecyber.com).

Lifelight Smart Wings

It's like you never left Hooters, huh? At least you kept those bright orange booty shorts as a souvenir. These veggie "chicken" wings are low in fat and high in protein. Available in Buffalo and Honey BBQ (lightlife.com).

Best Transition "Ribs"

Swap that

Old-fashioned barbecue ribs

for this

MorningStar Farms Hickory BBQ Riblets

The McRib is back! Not the one sold periodically at the Golden Arches. I'm talking about the most succulent ribs you've ever eaten, without the gristle. These look and taste just as meaty and rich as real ribs, with a seasoned BBQ sauce for flavor. Make sure you have some hand wipes nearby—things are about to get messy (morning starfarms.com).

> *These babies are prepackaged in little plastic bags for portion control. Pop them on a bun for a quick afternoon snack.*

Swap that ᘛᘛᘛ

Asian ribs

ᘛᘛᘛ *for this*

Vegetarian Plus Vegan Citrus Sparerib Cutlets

For some Asian persuasion, try these cutlets, which are soaked in a plum-wine garlic sauce. They're not the type you eat with your hands, but toss them in stir-fries or noodle dishes, and you'll croon. There is a reason they are Vegetarian Plus's bestselling product (vegeusa.com).

Deli Slices

Swap that ᘛᘛᘛ

Deli meat slices

ᘛᘛᘛ *for this*

Tofurky Meatless Deli Slices

Thin meatless slices that beef up any sandwich (pun intended). Tofurky offers a handful of flavor-packed varieties that are all made with nutritious ingredients and no GMOs. Available in flavors such as Pepperoni, Oven Roasted, Peppered, and Hickory Smoked (tofurky.com).

KIM'S PICK: The Cranberry and Stuffing Deli Slices are my all-time favorite—it's like eating Thanksgiving leftovers whenever you damn well please.

Best Variety of Vegan Deli Meats

Yves Deli Slices

You could make a sandwich every day of the week and never eat the same slice twice. That's because Yves delivers with seven savory, meatless varieties. Available in Bologna, Ham, Turkey, Salami, Pepperoni, Roast Without the Beef, and Smoked Chicken (yvesveggie.com).

Lightlife Smart Deli Baked Ham

Warning: this can get addictive. You add a few slices to a wrap, then you work them into a grilled cheese, and next thing you know, you're hoarding them in your purse and hiding them from your roommate. Everything in moderation, babe (lightlife.com).

Field Roast Deli Slices

From the same company that makes the most amazing meat sausages that have ever graced my lips, these charcuterie-style deli slices aren't so bad either. Available in Lentil Sage, Wild Mushroom, and Smoked Tomato (fieldroast.com).

Tuna

Tired of contributing to the overfishing of our seas? Ever since commercial fishing techniques were launched in the 1950s, the number of bluefin tuna has decreased by 97 percent. Yeah, almost the entire species. Thanks to our sushi obsession, chances are the wild bluefin tuna will go extinct by 2012. Do you want to be responsible for that? Enjoy a tunaless sandwich.

Swap that ᴕᴕᴕᴕ

Tuna salad

ᴕᴕᴕᴕ *for this*

Dixie Diner Tuna (Not!) Salad Mix

Just add a little water and vegan mayo, and voilà! (I add a little Follow Your Heart vegan mayo to get this mix nice and creamy.) You would think a fake tuna would be filled with gross ingredients, but there's nothing weird going on here—just some spices, veggie protein, and soy flour. It has a moist flavor without tasting too fishy, and it's delicious in a salad or on a fresh baguette with tomato slices and fresh basil (dixiediner.com).

Swap that ⟿

Canned tuna

⟿ *for this*

May Wah Vegetarian Tuna

A great alternative for traditional tuna in a can, this soy-based "tuna" with vegetarian seasonings has a shredded consistency that looks and feels like the real thing (vegieworld.com).

Vegetarian Plus Vegan Tuna Rolls

Vegan tuna made with soy and seaweed extract. Tasty on a whole-wheat bagel or to add protein to a salad (vegeusa.com).

Seafood

Swap that ⟿

Van de Camp's Frozen Seafood

⟿ *for this*

Sophie's Kitchen Seafood

Sophie's Kitchen was a father's answer to the problem of giving his daughter her favorite food after discovering she had a seafood allergy.

And now, it's all the answer I need. I will say I had serious hesitations about trying vegan seafood. Frankly, it freaked me the eff out. But Sophie's goods have the right texture and don't taste fishy *at all*. The shrimp and calamari even look spot-on (go ahead, analyze it), which is tough to pull off. Everything is GMO-free, with little to no saturated fat. Sophie's also donates 5 percent of net profits to support ocean species and habitat. Look for the Breaded Vegan Shrimp (gluten-free), Vegan Calamari, Vegan Prawn (gluten-free), Vegan Shrimp (gluten-free), Vegan Squid Ring (gluten-free), and Vegan Breaded Fish Fillet (sophieskitchen.net).

KIM'S PICK: Breaded fish fillets—they taste like chicken patties.

Vegetarian Plus Vegan Shrimp

These versatile vegan shrimp look and taste like the real thing, with coloring for effect. Add to salads, pasta dishes, and stir-fries or serve up as a shrimp cocktail (vegeusa.com).

Condiment Swaps

Hollah! Vegan Staple

Butter

If you're a baking whore, then butter is a tough one to give up as you make the transition to a plant-based diet. But seriously, bitches, it's foul. Butter contains not one, but two ingredients that make your cholesterol go haywire: dietary cholesterol and saturated fat. Vegan butters aren't free of saturated fat, but they contain about half the amount in every tablespoon. Dietary cholesterol, on the other hand, is exclusive to animal products. Give yourself a pat on the back. No more than 200 milligrams of cholesterol are recommended each day to stay healthy—butter delivers 33 milligrams in just one tablespoon! Hello, are you trying to put your heart through the ringer?! I hate to be the one to break it to you, but heart disease is the number one killer of women in this country. Use your brain and make the swap to something healthier for your pies and pancakes.

Swap that

Land O' Lakes Butter

for this

Earth Balance Natural Buttery Spread

Hallelujah. Free of GMOs, trans fats, hydrogenated oils, and artificial ingredients, Earth Balance should be a prerequisite for every American. And it's really the only butter that vegans go bonkers for. Earth Balance comes in a tub just like mama's margarine, but it has a thicker, creamier consistency. It also comes in sticks, which makes it ideal for measuring while baking. Get it anyway you like it: Soy Free, Whipped, Soy Garden, Vegan Buttery Sticks, or Made with Olive Oil (earthbalancenatural.com).

Mayonnaise

Let go of that mayo. Though a fat spoonful of the white, creamy stuff may spell extra flavor, traditional mayonnaise delivers 100 calories—80 of

Healthy Butter Alternatives

Skip the butter altogether, and go for natural apple, pear, or cashew butter. It's yummy on pancakes, waffles, and even PB&J sandwiches.

which come from fat—in just one tablespoon. And you wonder why you're having problems buttoning up your jeans? True, vegan mayonnaise isn't much different in the calorie department, but it also isn't made with eggs or dairy products, nasty artificial dyes, sweeteners, or substitutes like the real thing is. If you just can't deny yourself a little mayo, stick with one that's better for you all around.

Swap that ⟿

Best Foods or Hellman's Real Mayonnaise

⟿ for this

*Follow Your Heart Vegenaise

Originally a California-based health-food store with a renowned café, Follow Your Heart has been making gluten-free vegan products,

Healthier Mayo Alternatives

You can add some extra kick to a wrap without smothering on the calories. Try swapping out mayo with plain soy or rice yogurt, Dijon mustard, pesto, hummus, or creamy pureed avocado.

including dressings, imitation cheese, mayo, and sauces, for more than three decades. Every mayo flavor is so rich and so creamy I could bathe in it, and it's almost too good to be an imitation. Available in Original, Grapeseed Oil, High Omega-3, Organic Original, and Reduced Fat Flaxseed and Olive Oil (followyourheart.com).

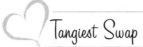 Tangiest Swap

*Nasoya Nayonaise

Though I don't like to play favorites—*cough, cough*—my son and I have a sweet spot for Nasoya Nayonaise. It has a tangy flavor with a hint of mustard and spreads smoothly because of its thinner texture (nasoya.com).

An asterisk (*) means the product is gluten-free.

*Spectrum Organics Light Canola Mayo

Want to maintain that girlish figure? Spectrum Organics' Light Canola Mayo only delivers a measly 35 calories per tablespoon. The vegan, gluten-free blend is made with expeller-pressed canola oil and spices, which makes it great for aioli too (spectrumorganics.com).

Ketchup

What could be so bad about something that comes from tomatoes? What our food-processing industry produces—that's what. Though ketchup is low in calories and fat-free, the large condiment peddlers load that bottle of red goodness with artificial sugars and sodium but disguise it as wholesome. Shake the guilt and dip your French fries in something better.

Swap that ⟿

Heinz Ketchup

⟿ *for this*

*Annie's Naturals Organic Ketchup

Annie Christopher's rich, savory ketchup tastes just like Heinz's, but there is one thing that definitely separates them—Annie's is made from simple, natural, organic ingredients, with no additives or preservatives (annies.com).

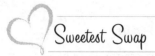 Sweetest Swap

*Krazy Ketchup

Made with 100 percent organic ingredients such as butternut squash, carrot, and sweet potato purees, this ketchup is like eating grown-up baby food. It has a tart, citrusy flavor that adults and kids love and is low in sodium (krazyketchup.org).

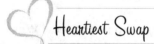 Heartiest Swap

*Organicville Organic Ketchup

This company makes more than a dozen products that fill my pantry, and its zesty organic ketchup always makes my shopping list. It has a filling, hearty taste, with no added sugar, and USDA-certified organic ingredients (organicvillefoods.com).

Gravy Mixes

I can still hear the voice in my head: "Kim, gone are the days where you could shower your mashed potatoes with gravy. Kiss good-bye the biscuits you threatened your mom she had to make or else you'd tell everyone in the neighborhood she was a sleaze. No, you're special now." You know what I tell that damn voice in my head now? You bet your ass I'm special. Now I

---

fat
fact

Have your utensils seen better days? Use ketchup to clean them up. The acid removes tarnish and shines up copper.

can still indulge in some of my most cherished comfort foods without sacrificing my beliefs.

*Road's End Organics Gravy Mixes

Road's End Organics knows what a girl with a conscience wants. Road's End Organics carries three different fat-free flavors that are all healthy for your bod and gluten-free. Treat your noodles, mashed potatoes, biscuits, sautéed seitan or tempeh, and Thanksgiving Tofurky to some fun. Available in Golden, Shiitake Mushroom, and Savory Herb (edwardandsons.com).

♡ *Best Swap for Holiday Cookin'*

Swap that ᴑᴑᴑᴑᴑ

McCormick Gravy Mixes

ᴑᴑᴑᴑᴑ *for this*

*Leahey Gravy Mixes

Leahey's Gravy Mixes have a thick base and come in a variety of savory flavors that complement any hearty dish. Choose from Creamy, Mushroom, No Beef Brown, No Beef Mexican Style, and No Chicken Golden, and the same lineup in gluten-free. If you can't make up your mind, try either of the Gravy Sampler Packs (leaheyfoods.com).

Worcestershire Sauce

Popularized in the mid-1800s by two dispensing chemists, Worcestershire sauce has long been popular for giving meat and fish a robust bite. But there are a few things you may care to know if you're introducing it to your vegan kitchen. One, it contains anchovies (I just threw up in my mouth). And, according to *Big Secrets* author William Poundhouse, beef extract and pork liver are common ingredients, though you won't find them in the list. Maybe that's what they mean by "natural flavorings." Natural, my ass. Since Worcestershire sauce belongs in every meatless kitchen, it's time to find one sans the corn syrup and roadkill.

*The Wizard's Organic Vegan Worcestershire Sauce

Get saucy with the Wizard's potent Worcestershire sauce, made with zesty organic tamarind, chili pepper, shiitake mushrooms, and soy. If gluten has got you down, try the organic, gluten-free flavor, which has a sweet kick (edwardandsons.com).

⇒ *A tough find in grocery stores, so buy online to save yourself some time.*

Swap that ⟿

⟿ *for this*

Annie's Naturals Organic Worcestershire Sauce

Annie's heady blend is balanced by hints of organic molasses and aromatic herbs, without the nasty, fishy anchovies (annies.com).

Pasta Sauce

Three Cheese, Italian Sausage, Creamy Alfredo, Mini Meatball. No, these aren't the meatheads on the Jersey Shore. This is the crap you're pouring all over that hefty helping of refined, starchy, white pasta. If you are trying to bulk up for the NFL, then by all means slurp it down, sister. But the pasta sauces you're finding on the shelves at your friendly major grocer are filled with empty calories, fat, sodium, and sugar. Skip the creamy, cheesy, meaty junk, and look for some of these healthier pasta sauces (and for the love of weight loss, please stick with whole-wheat pasta).

*Organicville Organic Pasta Sauce

Organicville's herb-infused Tomato Basil is made with 100 percent extra virgin olive oil, agave nectar, and organic tomatoes, basil, onions, garlic, and oregano. Also available in Marinara, Portabella, and Italian Herb (organicvillefoods.com).

*Amy's Premium Organic Pasta Sauce

Perfect for good ole-fashioned family cooking, Amy's simple pasta sauces are free of dairy, lactose, soy, tree nuts, gluten, and nasty ingredients. For those looking to cut their sodium, Amy's also offers lower-sodium versions of its traditional Tomato Basil and Family Marinara sauces (amys.com).

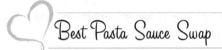 Best Pasta Sauce Swap

Lucini Italia Pasta Sauces

Lucini Italia's authentic Italian sauces are a gourmet upgrade from your everyday store-bought canned sauces. Each fancy-schmancy variety is handcrafted with hearty plum tomatoes, fresh herbs, and premium extra virgin olive oil, no added sugar or artificial ingredients. Vegan varieties are available in Hearty Artichoke Tomato, Sicilian Olive and Wild Caper, Spicy Tuscan Tomato, and Tuscan Marinara with Roasted Garlic (lucini.com).

KIM'S PICK: Tomato Basil has a fresh basil taste that wakes up a simple pasta dish. I stock my pantry with this stuff, so there is never fear of running out.

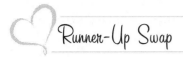

Cucina Antica Tomato Sauces

If your sauce style is more mom-and-pop, look no further than Cucina Antica's all-natural sauces made with imported plum tomatoes from southern Italy. The family-owned company has been making wannabe cooks say "Grazie" for generations. Like Lucini, it also leans on the gourmet side and isn't too chunky. Vegan varieties are available in Garlic Marinara and Tomato Basil (cucina-antica.com).

Trader Giotto's Pasta Sauce

Trader Joe's private Italian label, Trader Giotto's features a line of gourmet-style pasta sauces that really don't need any extra flavoring. Just heat and drizzle over pasta. Available in Tomato Basil Marinara (also in organic) and Roasted Garlic (traderjoes.com).

Soy Sauce

Leave it to us to cheapen a Chinese specialty with takeout packets and bottles of sodium overkill. The crap we've come to know as "soy sauce" is actually synthesized from hydrolyzed vegetable protein (HVP) and then mixed with hydrochloric acid. Oh, and they're not done. Manufacturers then add caramel coloring, preservatives, salt, high-fructose corn syrup, and refined sugars to pump up the flavor. Trust me, bitches, this wasn't the Asian way. When getting your soy-sauce fix, look for naturally fermented or brewed soy products that are made from non-GMO soybeans and do not contain HVP or artificial coloring. "Lite" versions will contain less sodium too.

Swap that ∽∽∽

Kikkoman Soy Sauce

∽∽∽ for this

San-J Organic Shoyu Naturally Brewed Soy Sauce

Brewed with soybeans and wheat for up to six months, this all-natural soy sauce is your pantry's BFF. It's pretty easy to find in stores and has a flavor similar to soy sauce in those little packets you find in Chinese restaurants, but without all the MSG and artificial preservatives (san-j.com).

*San-J Organic Tamari Gluten-Free Soy Sauce

Naturally brewed soy sauce made without the wheat. Available in the following certified gluten-free varieties: Regular, Organic, Reduced Sodium, and Organic Reduced Sodium (san-j.com).

Healthiest and Lightest Swap

*Coconut Secret Raw Coconut Aminos Soy-Free Seasoning Sauce

Founded by a brother-and-sister duo on a mission to find low-glycemic products for their diabetic parents, Coconut Secret makes products from the nutrient-rich "sap" from the coconut tree. Not a fan of sap? Consider this: coconut sap is actually a solid source of seventeen amino acids, plus minerals and vitamins. One hundred percent organic and certified by the USDA. A kitchen staple for any health nut (iherb.com).

Hollah! Vegan Staple

Best All-Around Swap

Braggs All Natural Liquid Aminos All-Purpose Seasoning

My go-to for almost every dish, Braggs is a versatile, certified non-GMO soy-sauce alternative that contains more than sixteen amino acids and only a percentage of the sodium. It's light, but without sacrificing the flavor (bragg.com).

Teriyaki and Asian Sauces

You can hate me for saying it, but if it's a sauce and it's in a bottle, it probably isn't good for you—especially if it's teriyaki sauce. There, I suck. The stuff that passes for traditional teriyaki sauce in the United States is filled with MSG, high-fructose corn syrup, modified starches, caramel coloring, and "natural flavors." Whatever the hell that means.

In the United States, 92 percent of soybeans are genetically modified, meaning they contain an evil gene that makes them resistant to pesticides and herbicides. By definition, the organic label means a food or product cannot contain GMOs. So do me a favor. Buy organic soy sauce.

Swap that ~~~~~

~~~~~ for this

Soy Vay Sauces

Soy Vay's versatile teriyaki sauces and marinades knock it right out of the park. They are the perfect mix of sweet and savory and have little sesame seeds that float at the top just begging me to eat them. (Oh, don't act like you're not so easily impressed.) All of the sauces are made with wholesome ingredients and are awesome for dipping. No preparation is needed for marinades—just coat vegetables right before cooking or toss on right before serving. Available in Wasabi Teriyaki, Veri Veri Teriyaki, Island Teriyaki, and Toasted Sesame Dressing and Marinade (soyvay.com).

Tamari and Shoyu

Here's how to tell these authentic Japanese soy sauces apart. Made from whole soybeans, sea salt, and water, *tamari* is commonly used for longer cooking methods, such as stews, soups, marinades, and baking. Substitute wheat for water in those ingredients, and you have *shoyu*. Used more often as an all-purpose cooking and table condiment, shoyu delivers a subtle flavor that doesn't overpower stir-fries, sauces, and vegetables.

Swap that ✐〜〜〜〜

Plum sauce

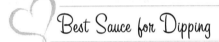 〜〜〜〜 **for this**

Lee Kum Kee Plum Sauce

Lee Kum Kee is your one-stop shop for savory sauces fit for veggie stir-fries, rice, or noodles, but the Plum Sauce is unmatched. Preserved Chinese plums, ginger, and chilies give it a rich, divine flavor (us.lkk.com).

Best Sauce for Dipping

*Premier Japan Hoisin Sauce

Premier Japan prides itself on its USDA-certified organic sauces made from naturally brewed soy sauces flavored with ginger, sesame, miso, or wasabi. The Hoisin Sauce is ideal for dipping anything from veggie pot stickers to spring rolls. Vegan varieties are also available in Teriyaki Sauce and Ginger Tamari (edwardandsons.com).

Trader Joe's Island Soyaki Teriyaki Marinade

A versatile marinade that will take over any dish. Pan-grill some assorted veggies on the stovetop with a few tablespoons of Soyaki and serve over brown rice. If there is any left over, save it for lunch the next day. Never gets old (traderjoes.com).

Barbecue Sauce

Want a sugar rush? Just dunk that Tofurky dog in some BBQ sauce. Heinz BBQ boasts smoke flavoring, brown sugar, and some more sugar. And taking the cake, KC Masterpiece's Hickory Brown Sugar BBQ Sauce contains sugar, high-fructose corn syrup and brown sugar and is finished off with caramel coloring and salt. Hell, why don't you just eat a few Fudgesicles, fatty?! These healthier, vegan BBQ sauces get their rich flavor from spices and herbs rather than sugar overkill.

*Annie's Naturals Hot Chipotle BBQ Sauce

You don't have to be a meat freak to appreciate Annie's smoky BBQ sauce, which packs some heat thanks to organic chipotle peppers (annies.com).

*Follow Your Heart Mild Balsamic Barbecue Sauce

Aged balsamic vinegar gives this hearty BBQ sauce a nice bite (followyourheart.com).

Hollah! Vegan Staple

Cooking Broth

Here's a nice story to share with your kids before bed. Meat broth is made by simmering bones or leftover cooked meat—all that delicious flavor in their soup comes from the cartilage and connective tissue of their favorite barnyard animal. See if that touching bedtime tale puts the kiddos soundly to sleep. Prepackaged broths and meat stocks also contain MSG and autolyzed yeast extract—two ingredients your body would rather do without. Ya heard me?

A broth should be a staple in any kitchen, especially in a vegan one, since it's great for adding flavor to rice and grain dishes. So look for broths that are certified organic, all-natural, and light on sodium. Swanson Vegetable Broth contains 940 milligrams of sodium in one cup, compared to 550 milligrams for the Swanson certified organic variety. Sodium is not bad for us—in fact, our bodies need it—but there is more than enough added to processed foods to preserve them longer and add nice flavor. No need to add more.

Swap that ∿∿∿

Swanson Vegetable Broth

∿∿∿ for this

*Pacific Natural Foods Organic Vegetable Broth

Vegan and gluten-free, Pacific's veggie broth is a light mixture of organic celery, carrots, tomatoes, garlic, onions, leeks, and spices. It's my go-to for every homemade dish and adds a nice subtle flavor to soups and rice dishes. You can also use it to replace water in any dish, since it's not too thick (pacificfoods.com).

Swap that ∿∿∿

Meat bouillon cubes

∿∿∿ for this

*Edward & Sons Natural Bouillon Cubes

Edward & Sons' Swiss-made Not-Chick'n and Not-Beef Bouillon Cubes are higher in fat and sodium, but as long as you use them in moderation, they will rock your world. Just drop them in the cooking water when making grains, quinoa, or soups, and the flavor takes over from there. They also carry Low-Sodium Veggie Cubes that boast only 125 milligrams of sodium (edwardandsons.com).

Rapunzel Vegan Vegetable Bouillon Cubes

Awesome for seasoning grains and soups, Rapunzel GMO-free bouillon is superlow in sodium (only 101 grams) and made from organic

If a recipe calls for beef broth, just swap it out for vegetable broth at a 1 to 1 ratio. You can also substitute 1 vegetable bouillon cube mixed with 1 cup of boiling water. And if you've been too lazy to hit up the grocery store—no sweat. Go for 1 tablespoon of soy sauce plus enough water to make 1 cup.

carrots, onions, celery, parsley, turmeric, and mace. Choose from three different options: Regular with Sea Salt, With Herbs, and No Salt Added (truefoodsmarket.com).

*Seitenbacher Vegetable Broth and Seasoning

Imported from Germany, Seitenbacher's broth is gluten-free with no stinkin' MSG. Unique ingredients such as lovage, paprika, and nutmeg make this one extra special (store.veganessentials.com).

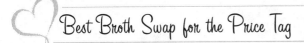

Best Broth Swap for the Price Tag

*Trader Joe's Organic Vegetable Broth

Leave it to Trader Joe's to offer a delicious, savory broth at a super-reasonable price. Its Hearty Vegetable Broth doesn't skimp on flavor, nor does it overdose on salt. But if you're watching your sodium intake, it also offers a low-sodium variety (traderjoes.com).

Cooking Sauces

Unless veggies drive you absolutely wild, it's always good to have a solid stash of cooking sauces in the pantry for waking up noodles, tofu, and meat alternatives. Not the artificial-ingredient overkill in packaged marinades and sauces . . . I mean, healthy sauces. They spice up even the blandest dishes and give them that gourmet twist.

*Spicy Nothings

Gourmet Indian curry sauces made with wholesome ingredients and no pastes or powders. No artificial flavors, preservatives, or MSG. Try the Spinach and Cream Curry Simmer Sauce and Classic Curry Simmer Sauce (spicynothings.com).

♡ Best Curry Swap

Swap that ∽∽∽

Yellow or red curry

∽∽∽ for this

*Mike's Organic Curry Love Curries

Seriously, where the hell have you been all my life? These certified organic, gluten-free curries are ready-made, so you just heat and eat, baby. If you're cooking for one, you won't use the whole jar (well, let's hope not, Miss Piggy). Just make sure you tighten the lid and then, next time, pour some curry love all over your rice and veggies for dinner. For yellow curry, use Blissful Banana Ginger or Luscious Yellow Thai; for red curry, Passion Red Thai or Tantalizing Tomato Coconut (mycurrylove.com).

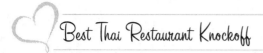
Best Thai Restaurant Knockoff

*Tasty Bite Cooking Sauces

The Pad Thai and Satay Partay are both copies of the classics and ideal for marinating tofu, seitan, tempeh, and veggies—try it with Dixie Diner's Chicken (Not!) Breast. Just toss over noodles and serve. Also available in Good Korma, with cashews, coconut, and spices (tastybite.com).

Pestos and Tapenades

Must haves for every kitchen, pestos and tapenades make good dipping sauces for a quick snack or appetizer. They can be used as flavorful spreads on sandwiches, crusty bread, bruschetta, or crackers, and pesto is great for mixing with pasta, meat alternatives, and grilled veggies.

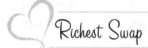
Richest Swap

*Meditalia Basil Pesto

Produced in Israel by a co-op composed of Israelis, Arabs, and other close neighbors, this vegan pesto has a fresh olive oil and basil flavor. Also available are various olive, pepper, and tomato tapenades (peace works.com).

KIM'S PICK: Roasted Eggplant Tapenade—it's freakin' divine!

Swap that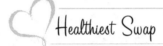

Classico Pesto Sauce

for this

Radici of Tuscany Vegan Basil Pesto

The freshest, most authentic, basil*iest* pesto in a jar. The distributor, Ritrovo, carries a line of heirloom products and ready-to-eat sauces that are 100 percent organic. You'll feel like you're rendezvousing in Italy (ritrovo.com).

Healthiest Swap

Living Tree Community Foods Tahinis, Olive Oils, and Nut Butters

Raw foodies go all whacky for these raw ("alive") organic oils and butters. Spread on flaxseed crackers or vegetable slices (livingtree community.com).

KIM'S PICK: Organic Walnut Pesto, a welcome change from the traditional pine nuts and basil pestos. It's thick and spreadable, with such a smooth nutty taste.

Simply Organic Sweet Basil Pesto Seasoning Mix

This easy-to-prepare mix is USDA-certified organic and tastes like fresh basil. Just mix with water and olive oil, then heat on the stovetop. Great with mashed potatoes, pasta, or on stuffed portobello mushrooms (simplyorganicfoods.com).

Seasonings

Vegetarian meat and tofu are easy to liven up with some hearty, fresh spices that bring worldly flavor into your kitchen. Sloppy joes aren't even out of the question. Hey, you may be vegan, but you're not dead.

Fantastic World Foods Mixes

Sourcing natural and organic ingredients from across the globe, Fantastic World Foods blends ethnic and regional cuisines for new appetites. Try the premade mixes in Tofu Scrambler, Vegetarian Chili, Vegan Taco Filling, Nature's Burger, and Vegan Sloppy Joe (fantasticfoods.com).

Nutritional Yeast

Similar in taste to the Aussie staple Vegemite, nutritional yeast is a vegan staple traditionally used to add some nutty, cheesy, creamy flavoring to foods. It's naturally low in fat and sodium and high in B vitamins, amino acids, and minerals. Here's the thing: you either love it or hate it. I happen to dig it. Nutritional yeast comes in a yellow powder or flake form. Sprinkle

Nutritional Yeast

Nutritional yeast is made by fermenting yeast with a blend of sugar-cane and beet molasses.

it over popcorn, potatoes, or tofu, and use it to make soups, gravy, and sauces richer.

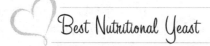 Best Nutritional Yeast

*NOW Nutritional Yeast Flakes

GMO-free dried yeast in flake form that is used to add a cheesy flavor to sauces. NOW's yeast flakes are fortified with additional B vitamins, which are good for the brain (sprinkle a few tablespoons into a glass of soy milk for a healthy boost; nowfoods.com).

*Organic Gourmet European Nutritional Yeast Extract Savory Spread

This spread has a thicker consistency, so it's best for jazzing up soups, stews, and gravies. Gluten-free and low in salt (organic-gourmet.com).

Red Star Nutritional Yeast

Used more as a cheese substitute, Red Star is great for making doughs and breads (redstaryeast.com).

Hummus

If there is any food I will tell you to shovel down your throat like cake, it's hummus. A popular Mediterranean food, hummus is a dip or spread made by cooking up mashed chickpeas (garbanzos) and blending them with tahini, olive oil, lemon juice, salt, and garlic. Chickpeas are a good source of protein, and overall hummus is high in vitamins B6 and C, iron, and folate. Try it with pita bread or use it as a veggie dip.

Trader Joe's Organic Hummus Dip

This one's destined to be a classic. It tastes like it's homemade and is great with chips and pita crisps. Try it in Roasted Garlic or Mediterranean (traderjoes.com).

Wildwood Organic Probiotic Hummus

Wildwood offers a wide variety of veggie products from sprouted tofu to probiotic soymilk. Because it emphasizes beneficial nondairy cultures, this company also pumps its hummus with probiotics to promote healthy digestion. No matter which flavor you go with, it's so creamy and bursting with flavor. Available in Classic, Roasted Red Pepper, Spicy Cayenne, and Low Fat Classic (pulmuonewildwood.com).

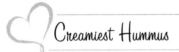
Creamiest Hummus

Cedar's Simply Delicious Hommus

The man behind this magic has a deep passion for Mediterranean foods, and it shows. The Organic Original, Organic Garlic Lovers, and Original Hommus Tahini are fan favorites, but it comes in a number of different varieties (cedarsfoods.com).

KIM'S PICK: Organic Garlic Lovers—perfect without an overbearing garlic bite.

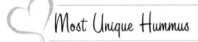
Most Unique Hummus

Haig's Delicacies Hummus

Mediterranean mezé from a family recipe, this one is on the whipped side with a zesty lemon zing, making it stand out among other brands. Try the Garbanzo Bean Mezé Hummus or Garbanzo Bean Mezé with Roasted Red Peppers (haigsdelicacies.com).

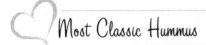
Most Classic Hummus

Athenos Hummus

Found at any major grocery chain, this one's stronger in flavor and not as creamy, but Skinny Bitches will love the light texture and classic taste. Available in Original, Roasted Garlic, and Artichoke and Garlic (athenos.com).

Dips

Did you ever read the back of the dip label before you dipped that chip? It may taste like French onion heaven, but dips are typically packing tons o' sour cream and mayonnaise, which doesn't just mean you're eating animals—you're also loading up on saturated fats and cholesterol. But let's be real. You're dipping days are not behind you. Just because you've gone veg, doesn't mean you're done jazzing up chips, crackers, and raw veggies with creamy goodness. What else are you going bring to the next vegan tailgate party? (Yeah right.) If you're big on dipping, stick with the healthier versions without all the fat and cholesterol. Companies like Wayfare make their "cheese" spreads from oatmeal. Totally kewl.

Swap that ⟶

French onion dip

⟵ for this

Simply Organic French Onion Dip

If you're entertaining and want to serve vegan snacks without looking like a selfish a-hole, these dips will fool anybody. They are easy to prepare; just mix with vegan sour cream or soy yogurt (simplyorganic foods.com).

Swap that 〰〰〰

Marie's Creamy Dill Dip

〰〰〰 *for this*

Simply Organic Creamy Dill Dip

A spunky combo of garlic, onion, celery seed, and dill that tastes great with pita chips, on a baked potato, or as a sandwich spread (simply organicfoods.com).

Swap that 〰〰〰

Pâté

〰〰〰 *for this*

Tartex Vegan Pâté

Pâté is a mixture of ground meat and animal fat minced into a spreadable paste. People actually eat it. With their mouth. Gag me. With a spoon. This vegan version is an import from Germany made with veggies, organic potato starch, nonhydrogenated oils, and herbs. It's rich, "meaty," and yet so light on a baguette, French bread, or crackers. My French mother-in-law has been sending this to me for the past decade. Available in Original, Mushroom, and Herb Meadow (tartex.com).

Swap that

Cheese spread

for this

Wayfare "We Can't Say It's Cheese" Dips and Spreads

Certified gluten-free without wheat, soy, GMOs, or trans fats, these faux cheese dips and spreads are made with whole-grain oatmeal. Choose from dips in Cheddar-Style and Mexi-Cheddar Style or spreads in Cheddar-Style and Hickory-Smoked Cheddar-Style (wayfarefoods.com).

KIM'S PICK: The richest, most cheddarlike is the Hickory-Smoked Cheddar-Style.

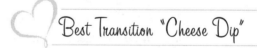 Best Transition "Cheese Dip"

Swap that

Nacho cheese dip

for this

Food for Lovers Vegan Queso

This spicy vegan cheesy sauce kind of took me by surprise—it tastes just like the Tostitos Salsa Con Queso I used to pour all over my nachos in my twenties like I had Victoria Beckham's metabolism. To get the full effect, heat it up in a microwave-safe bowl for 1 to 2 minutes, stirring every 30 seconds, and serve (it's much better when heated). It's thick and creamy for dipping chips, or use it as a topping for any Mexican-style dish. The "cheese" is made with nutritional yeast and contains no fat, soy, or nuts (food-for-lovers.com).

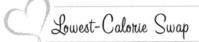

Lowest-Calorie Swap

*Nacho Mom's Ultimate Vegan Queso

Named "Best New Product" by *VegNews* magazine, this jar of cheesy goodness is another favorite for baked potatoes, vegan chili cheese dogs, and nachos. Free of gluten and soy, and only 160 calories in the entire jar! Available in Ultimate Vegan Queso, Fire Roasted Queso, and Voodoo Queso (fatgoblin.com).

> *If you're a fan of nutritional yeast, then try this queso. It has a yeasty flavor and a sharpness to it that some vegans swear by.*

Swap that ⟳⟳⟳⟳

Tostitos Chunky Salsa

⟲⟲⟲⟲ *for this*

365 Organic Salsa

This Whole Foods salsa is chunky and filling; it will tide you over until the next meal or let you entertain guests for a cheap price. It comes in mild, medium, and hot depending on how much of a wuss you are (wholefoodsmarket.com).

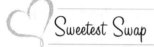 *Sweetest Swap*

Organicville Organic Salsa

Available in mild or medium, Organicville Salsa is sweetened with agave nectar, which pairs really well with the savory flavor of tomatoes (no stinkin' high-fructose corn syrup here, missy; organicville foods.com).

Fruit Spreads

Were you hoping for real fruit in that spread? You're adorable. Most fruit jellies and jams are just sugar with some artificial fruit flavoring and a smidgen of the real thing. Let's go to the tapes, shall we? Just one tablespoon of Smucker's Jam contains 50 calories and a whopping 12 grams of sugar. Here are a few rad fruit spreads that are naturally sweetened with organic ingredients and contain half the sugar and calories.

Swap that ∿∿∿⟶

Smucker's Jam

⟵∿∿∿ for this

Trader Joe's Fruit Spreads

Give me that sweet, that tasty, that sticky stuff. TJ's organic fruit spreads contain only the fruit and vitamin C and, although thinner in consistency, they're not runny. The texture feels just like the stuff you grew up on. Available in Strawberry, Apricot, Raspberry, Blueberry, and Superfruit (traderjoes.com).

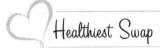 Healthiest Swap

Bionaturae Fruit Spreads

Made with organic apple juice concentrate and heirloom varieties of Italian fruit, Bionaturae's spreads are low in sugar, but no less sweet. Available in Apricot, Peach, Plum, Red Raspberry, Sicilian Orange, Sour Cherry, Strawberry, Wild Berry, Wild Blackberry, and Bilberry (bionaturae.com).

▸ *More fruity flavors than Baskin-Robbins!*

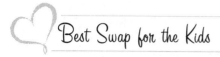

Best Swap for the Kids

Crofter's Organic Just Fruit Spreads

These are made with 100 percent fruit and sweetened with concentrated organic grape juice sourced from an Italian winemaker. Cheers to that. Available in Strawberry, Wild Blueberry, Raspberry, Apricot, Blackberry, Black Currant, and Superfruit (croftersorganic.com).

Most Unique Fruit Spread

Crofter's Superfruit Spreads

Everyone knows you get around, so why not embrace it with Crofter's four Superfruit spreads, sourced from around the globe. They are made with premium organic fruit, sweetened with fair-trade sugar, and pumped with antioxidants. Available in Asia (yumberries and raspberries), Europe (pomegranate and black currants blended with red grapes and morello cherries), North America (wild cranberries and blueberries blended with red grapes and morello cherries), and South America (maqui berries and passionfruit blended with red grapes and morello cherries; croftersorganic.com).

KIM'S PICK: I have a major crush on the Asia fruit spread, which has little chunks of raspberries that are bursting with flavor.

Nut Butters

If you ask me, peanut butter is one of life's most perfect foods. It livens up the nutritional count of food, it's high in protein, and it goes with just about everything. That is, when it doesn't go by the name of Jif or Skippy. Commercial brands jack up the sugar, hydrogenated vegetable oils, and mono- and diglycerides (which can come from animal fat). Today, you can find more pure, raw, and natural nut butters made from almonds, cashews, and sunflower seeds. Just stick to the Skinny Bitch way and aim for simple ingredients that you can recognize.

Trader Joe's Almond Butter

A food paste made from almonds, this almond butter is high in mono-unsaturated fats (same stuff that's in avocados) and a great source of fiber. Available in Almond Butter with Roasted Flaxseeds, Organic Creamy, Organic Crunchy, Organic Creamy Unsalted, and Organic Crunchy Unsalted (traderjoes.com).

Rejuvenative Foods Fresh Raw Almond Butter

Made from 100 percent fresh, raw organic almonds, this butter is freshly ground several times to maintain its "life energy." Whatever that means, I'm sold. In the refrigerated section (rejuvenative.com).

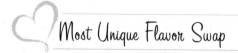

Most Unique Flavor Swap

Peanut Butter & Co. Gourmet Peanut Butter

So here's where I break my own rule. This peanut butters is not organic, but the flavors are mouthwatering, and the ingredients simple. Available in White Chocolate Wonderful, Dark Chocolate Dreams, Cinnamon Raisin Swirl, Smooth Operator, Mighty Maple, and Crunch Time (ilovepeanutbutter.com).

Tropical Traditions Organic Coconut Peanut Butter

Only two ingredients in this jar: organic Valencia peanuts and organic coconut (tropicaltraditions.com).

Swap that ᴑᴑᴑᴑᴑ

Jif Peanut Butter

ᴑᴑᴑᴑᴑ for this

O Organics Old Fashioned Creamy Peanut Butter

Just like the nostalgic peanut butter from our younger years, O Organics certified organic peanut butter is supergooey and buttery (safe way.com).

Organic NuttZo Omega-3 Multi-Nut Butter

A protein-packed peanut butter with organic hazelnuts, flax seeds, sunflower seeds, Brazil nuts, cashews, almonds, and Valencia peanuts. Stir it up before you refrigerate, so it doesn't harden (gonuttzo.com).

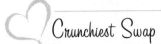 *Best Nut Butter for Cooking*

Sunland Organic Peanut Butter

Unique in its own right, Sunland's peanut butter isn't only marvelous on a PB&J. It's great in Asian cooking to make homemade peanut sauces. Available in different flavors: Creamy Cherry Vanilla, Chipotle Chile, Crunchy Chipotle Chile, Thai Ginger and Red Pepper, and Valencia Crunchy (sunlandinc.com).

KIM'S PICKS: The Thai Ginger and Red Pepper and Chipotle Chile varieties make a bomb pad thai.

Crunchiest Swap

Woodstock Farms Nut Butter

A natural line of nut butters perfect for every day. Varieties come in salted or unsalted, with tons of fresh, crunchy peanuts. Available in Organic Classic Peanut Butter (crunchy and smooth), Almond Butter (crunchy and smooth), Cashew Butter Unsalted, Tahini Unsalted, and Organic Raw Almond Butter (woodstock-farms.com).

Futters Nut Butter

A family-run, woman-owned business, Futters has a huge selection—practically any nut butter you can imagine—all with no gluten, salt, sugar, or trans fats. Available in Almond Butter, Macadamia Nut Butter, Brazil Nut Butter, Pistachio Nut Butter, Cashew Butter, Pumpkin Seed Butter, Hazelnut Butter, Sunflower Seed Butter, Almond Hazelnut Butter, and Walnut and Pecan Butter (futtersnutbutters.com).

Salad Dressing

Thanks to salad dressing, salads have gotten a bad rap for chicks trying to shed some pounds. French dressing packs a whopping 88 calories per tablespoon (and you drench your greens in it). Empty calories aside, even the more "simple" bottled dressings contain sugar, egg yolks, cheese, milk, disodium EDTA (yes, a nasty preservative), and artificial coloring. Though some of my all-time favorite vegan dressings aren't much lighter on the calories, they won't trash your health. Find your favorite.

Annie's Naturals Dressings

Annie's offers a knock-your-socks-off line of natural and organic dressings that are great on salads or as a mayo replacement on wraps, sandwiches, or veggie burgers. Gluten-free varieties are available. Try the Lite Goddess, Goddess, Shiitake and Sesame, Tuscany Italian, Woodstock, Fat Free Raspberry Balsamic Vinaigrette, Lite Herb Balsamic, and Fat Free Mango Vinaigrette. Organic vegan dressings are available in Pomegranate Vinaigrette, Asian Sesame, French, Goddess, Oil and Vinegar, Papaya Poppy Seed, Red Wine and Olive Oil Vinaigrette, and Roasted Garlic Vinaigrette (annies.com).

KIM'S PICKS: The Goddess dressing, a creamy tahini and lemon blend, is insane. The organic Asian Sesame is also a pleasure on steamed veggies or as a marinade (just ask my son).

*Spectrum Organics Organic Vegan Caesar Salad Dressing

Though the entire dressing line is clean and zesty, the gluten-free vegan Caesar is drool-worthy. If you decide to experiment with other dressings, read the ingredients closely, since some aren't vegan (spectrum organics.com).

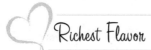

Richest Flavor

*Follow Your Heart Dressing

When everyone else zigs, Follow Your Heart zags. It avoids convention and flirts with original, distinctive organic and gluten-free dressing flavors that are lush and full-bodied. Available in Vegan Caesar, Vegan Thousand Island, Vegan Sesame Dijon, Vegan Creamy Garlic, Vegan Lemon Herb, Vegan Honey Mustard, Organic Balsamic Vinaigrette, and Organic Italian Vinaigrette, and Organic Miso Ginger. Drizzle on a veggie burger or a Tofurky club sandwich (followyourheart.com).

KIM'S PICKS: Thousand Island and Miso Ginger.

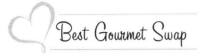
Best Gourmet Swap

Righteous Raspberry and Sweet Basil Dressing

This is the fancy stuff for salads. The fruit and herbs don't overpower one another for a sassy blend of sweet and savory. Guests think I'm some gourmet genius when I whip this stuff out at dinner. (Always present it in a bowl with a serving spoon, so nobody knows your secret. It's safe with me.) Good for your health and Mama Earth, Righteous all-natural dressings are also rich in omega-3s and make the perfect summer dressings (loverighteous.com).

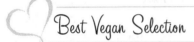
Best Vegan Selection

Newman's Own Salad Dressings

Newman's Own dressings are fairly natural and easy to get your hands on, available at any ole grocery-store chain. Vegan dressings are available in Organic Low Fat Asian, Organic Tuscan Italian, Lighten Up Balsamic Vinaigrette, Lighten Up Italian, Lighten Up Raspberry and Walnut, Lighten Up Red Wine Vinegar and Olive Oil, Lighten Up Roast Garlic Balsamic, Lighten Up Low Fat Sesame Ginger, and Olive Oil and Vinegar (newmansown.com).

KIM'S PICKS: Organic Tuscan Italian and the Lighten Up Low Fat Sesame Ginger.

Hollah! Vegan Staple

Oils and Vinegars

Woman, don't even think you can call yourself a cook without a good oil and a good vinegar in your arsenal. Unless you are trying to barbecue everything. For one, cooking oils are your BFF for baking, marinades, and stir-fries. Though canola oil is one of the more popular oils for cooking because of its neutral taste, I use, variously, grapeseed, extra virgin olive, safflower, and sunflower oil. Safflower and sunflower are great, because they can withstand high heat and have a very mild flavor, so they don't interfere with the dish. Vinegars get a thumbs-up because they can replace salt and give everything an extra bite. Apple cider, rice, balsamic, white-wine, and white vinegars are all versatile tools for everyday cooking.

Know your stuff

Some oils—walnut, flaxseed, and hempseed—work best for already cooked foods like salads, pasta, and grilled veggies. But I wouldn't recommend pan-grilling a veggie burger in them. Look for the key words "expeller," "cold-pressed," and "organic" when buying serving oils. This will get you the best in quality and flavor.

Spectrum Organic Cooking Oils

The nation's leader in organic, expeller-pressed culinary oils, Spectrum doesn't come up short. It employs natural processing methods, and its packaging is designed to protect the essential fatty acids in every bottle. You can get almond, apricot kernel, avocado, canola, grapeseed, peanut, safflower, sesame, sunflower, and walnut oils in refined, unrefined, organic, and high-heat varieties. For greasing pans or cookie sheets, try Spectrum's Canola Baking Spray Oil with Flour, which contains no chlorofluorocarbons (no good for Mama Earth). Also available in Canola Spray Oil, Grapeseed Spray Oil, and Coconut Spray Oil (spectrumorganics.com).

Trader Joe's Oils and Vinegars

These oils are what Trader Joe's stands for: cheap and accessible without sacrificing quality. Available in 100% Italian Extra Virgin Olive Oil Cold Pressed, Spanish Extra Virgin Olive Oil, Trader Giotto's Extra Virgin Olive Oil Cold Pressed, Trader Joe's 100% Canola Oil, and Grapeseed Oil. Vinegars are available in Unfiltered Apple Cider Vinegar and Red Wine Vinegar (traderjoes.com).

Eden Organic Oils and Vinegars

Eden's oils come in tinted bottles to protect the quality of the oil from light. Available in Olive Oil Extra Virgin Spanish, Safflower Oil, Sesame Oil Extra Virgin, Soybean Oil, and Toasted Sesame Oil. Vinegars are Organic Apple Cider Vinegar and Red Wine Vinegar (edenfoods.com).

Napa Valley Naturals Oils, Vinegars, and Cooking Wines

Frankly, they had me at "wine." This small, family-owned business makes certified organic oils, vinegars, and even artisan California cooking wines in dozens of varieties. And you can feel good bringing it into your kitchen—10 percent of proceeds are donated to environmental preservation, sustainable agriculture practices, and hunger prevention. Try the Extra Virgin Organic Olive Oil, which is cold-pressed and delivers a medium-bodied flavor that complements any dish (napavalleytrading.com).

Lucini Italia Oils and Vinegars

Lucini's Premium Select Extra Virgin Olive Oil is made from hand-picked Italian olives, cold pressed within twenty-four hours. Also try the Pinot Noir Italian Wine Vinegar and Savory Fig Balsamico Artisan Vinegar (lucini.com).

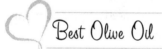 Best Olive Oil

O Olive Oil Oils and Vinegars

O Olive Oil makes the absolute best olive oil. My favorite flavors are the O Meyer Lemon Olive Oil and the O Ultra Premium Extra Virgin Olive Oil. For vinegars that stand out, O's rice and wine vinegars are flavor kickers. The Yuzu Rice Vinegar is sweet and tart with citrusy hints of Meyer lemon, lime, and tangerine. Also try the Champagne Vinegar (O's top-selling vinegar), which brings a crisp, bubbly accent to a vinaigrette dressing. The Cabernet Vinegar is aged in oak barrels under the sun and carries deep cherry notes. Drizzle any over salads with olive oil or add to Asian sauces and marinades (ooliveoil.com).

La Tourangelle Artisan Oils

La Tourangelle produces a range of nutty varieties ideal for salads, veggies, pasta, and hummus dishes. Choose from Roasted Pecan, Roasted Pistachio, 100% Organic Sunflower, Roasted Walnut, Roasted Almond, and Roasted Hazelnut (latourangelle.com).

CHAPTER

10

Dry Goods Swaps

Pasta

You won't catch me bitchin' about pasta carbs. My beef with pasta is that the average American consumes about twenty pounds of it every year—and most of it is the white, refined crap. Standard pastas are made with refined wheat flour that goes through intensive processing, which strips away all the germ and bran and leaves only the starchy stuff. So what you're left with basically has no nutritional value. None.

Speaking of what's in the stuff, shoppers should check for hidden ingredients such as whey, eggs, and butter. The biggest culprit is obviously egg noodles. Though most boxed and store-bought pasta is vegan—praise the vegan gods—some manufacturers such as Pennsylvania Dutch and Mueller's are all up on eggs, because they make pasta nice and fluffy.

Make the switch to 100 percent whole-grain, brown-rice, and oat-flour pastas, which have more fiber and take longer to digest, so you won't feel the need to stuff your face every ten minutes. The healthier versions also have more protein and are lower in calories. I'd chalk that one up as a win-win, sweetheart.

Trader Joe's Pasta

Trader Joe's signature line of pastas isn't only dirt cheap; it also beat out some pretty fancy brands in taste tests, like that of *New York* magazine. Available in Whole Wheat Spaghetti, Whole Wheat Pasta (penne and rotelle), Organic Brown Rice Spaghetti Pasta, and Organic Pasta Vegetable Radiatore (traderjoes.com).

*Bionaturae Pastas

Organic, authentic Italian pastas made from ingredients grown on small family farms. Available in Organic Gluten Free Fusilli, Penne Rigate, and Spaghetti (bionaturae.com).

*Tinkyada Pasta Joy Ready

Al dente pasta made from stone-ground rice that doesn't get that mushy texture. Certified organic and free of gluten and wheat. Try the White Rice Pasta Spaghetti Style, Brown Rice Pasta Shells with Rice Bran, Brown Rice Pasta Spaghetti Style, Spinach Spaghetti Style, Brown Rice Pasta Vegetable Spirals, Brown Rice Pasta (penne, elbow, and spirals), and Brown Rice Little Dreams with Rice Bran (tinkyada.com).

An asterisk (*) means the product is gluten-free.

*DeBoles Organic and All-Natural Pastas

DeBoles offers a great variety of different pasta shapes and flavors. My favorites are Spinach Fettuccine (made with Jerusalem artichoke flour), Whole Wheat Spaghetti Style, Whole Wheat Angel Hair, and Spinach Spaghetti Style. Also look for DeBoles gluten-free pastas in Rice Spaghetti Style, Whole Grain Spaghetti Style (made with rice and organic quinoa and amaranth flours; deboles.com).

*Ancient Harvest Quinoa Supergrain Pasta

Ancient Harvest's pastas are made with organic corn and quinoa flour in a gluten-free facility. Quinoa is an alkaline food that is a solid source of protein and promotes good health. Available in Garden Pagodas, Veggie Curls, Rotelle, Shells, Elbows, and Spaghetti Style (quinoa.net).

Noodles

Soba noodles, thin Japanese noodles, are traditionally used in hot and cold Thai and ethnic dishes. They are much better for you than the processed white crap, because they retain the nutrients in buckwheat and wheat flour. In fact, buckwheat is high in protein and fiber and contains all of the amino acids. Toss them with veggies and prepare with peanut or soy sauce. Udon—a thick wheat-flour noodle—is another popular noodle in Japanese cuisine that is usually served hot in noodle soups. Both pasta alternatives will give you some variety—just pick up a cookbook.

fat fact

Metal cans are still lined with a toxic chemical called BPA, which mimics your natural estrogen and makes your hormones go haywire. Even at low doses, it's been linked to some crazy shit, including cancer, infertility, birth defects, miscarriages, and Type II diabetes. Though we're fighting real hard for regulation to get it out of metal cans, many major manufacturers refuse to remove it. Protect yourself by looking for canned foods that are BPA-free.

Eden Organic Soba Noodles and Udon

Eden Organic offers a large selection of soba noodles and udon that make for lively soups and pad thai dishes. Available in a number of varieties and flavors, including Brown Rice Udon, Organic Kamut Soba, Organic Kamut Udon, Kuzu Pasta, Lotus Root Soba, Mugwort Soba, Mung Bean Pasta, Soba 100% Buckwheat, Organic Soba, Organic Spelt Soba, Organic Spelt Udon, Udon, Organic Udon 100% Whole Grain, Organic Wheat and Rice Udon, and Wild Yam Soba (edenfoods.com).

HakuBaku Authentic Japanese Noodles

Made in the Down Under from Australia's finest natural wheat with no artificial ingredients or added salt, this line of organic soba, somen (thinnest of all Japanese noodles), and udon noodles is kick-ass. Available in Organic Somen, Organic Soba, and Organic Udon (hakubaku.com).

Canned Beans

Cans of beans should be a staple in your pantry. They are great for adding flavor and protein to many dishes.

Trader Joe's Organic Beans

Available in Garbanzo Beans, Organic Kidney Beans, Organic Pinto Beans, White Kidney Beans, and Organic Black Beans (traderjoes.com).

Eden Organic Canned Beans

Eden stays true to its philosophy with a line of organic canned beans (in BPA-free cans) that are widely available in natural-foods stores across the country. Available in a few dozen varieties, including Black Turtle Beans, Dark Red Kidney Beans, Garbanzo Beans, Navy Beans, Pinto Beans, and Cannellini Beans (edenfoods.com).

365 Everyday Value Canned Beans

Whole Foods' signature brand, 365 Everyday Value, offers a great selection of canned beans at a price that's nice on the wallet. Available in Pinto, Garbanzo, Kidney, Black Beans, Black-Eyed Peas, Cannellini Beans, and selections with no added salt (wholefoodsmarket.com).

Eden Organic Canned Rice and Beans and Chilis

Mix it up with these BPA-free canned chilis and organic grain and bean combos to make a tasty side dish. Some of my favorites are Rice and Beans, Cajun Rice and Beans, Moroccan Rice and Beans, Curried Rice and Beans, Black Bean and Quinoa Chili, Great Northern Bean and Barley Chili, and Kidney Bean and Kamut Chili (edenfoods.com).

Canned Tomatoes

Although I'm a sucker for fresh farmers-market buys, I do love canned tomatoes. Why? Because you don't have to use them in a week and they are the foundation for almost every one of my most cherished recipes: spaghetti sauce, chili, and Italian casseroles. All you have to do is add some salt, pepper, onion, garlic, and spices to jazz up the flavor.

*Eden Organic Tomatoes

Eden packs its organic tomatoes in jars or cans with added spices and herbs, like roasted garlic and sweet basil. Plus, it offers you the option of no added salt. Choose from Crushed Tomatoes, Whole Roma Tomatoes, and Diced Tomatoes (edenfoods.com).

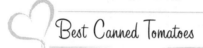

Best Canned Tomatoes

Muir Glen Organic Canned Tomatoes

Tomatoes grown in sunny California and combined with only wholesome, organic ingredients. Every variety is full-bodied and savory enough for any authentic Italian dish. Plus you can find them at any major grocer. Muir Glen also offers varieties with added Italian herbs, garlic, onion, and basil. Choose from Diced Tomatoes, Organic Tomato Sauce, and Organic Tomato Paste (muirglen.com).

Rao's Homemade Italian Peeled Tomatoes

Imported from Italy, and soaking in a tomato puree with basil leaf (raos.com).

O Organic Diced Tomatoes

Diced Tomatoes in Tomato Juice, Diced Tomatoes with Garlic, Basil, and Oregano, No Salt Diced Tomatoes, Whole Peeled Tomatoes in Tomato Juice, Tomato Paste (safeway.com).

Dried Beans and Lentils

Arrowhead Mills Beans and Lentils

Get your fill of protein and fiber with Arrowhead Mills' organic line of beans and lentils. Available in Green Lentils, Red Lentils, Green Split Peas, and Yellow Split Peas (arrowheadmills.com).

Soups

Premade soups are awesome to have on hand for chilly nights, when you don't have an extra minute to cook, when you're sick as a dog, or when you just feel like being a lazy ass. I like to keep a few healthy, hearty blends in the pantry for all of the above.

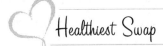

Healthiest Swap

Amy's Organics Soups

So little time, and so many to choose from. The queen of natural foods has one of the best selections of chunky soups known to woman. They are available in original, organic, and light-in-sodium varieties and are popping up left and right at everyday grocers. Vegan varieties are available in Alphabet Soup, Black Bean Vegetable, Chunky Vegetable, Indian Dal Golden Lentil, No Chicken Noodle Soup, Lentil, Lentil Vegetable, Fire Roasted Southwestern Vegetable, Indian Dal Curried Lentil, Hearty Spanish Rice and Red Bean, Minestrone, Thai Coconut

(Tom Kha Prak), Butternut Squash, Split Pea, French Country Vegetable, Hearty Rustic Italian Vegetable, Pasta and 3 Bean, Vegetable
Barley, and Tuscan Bean and Rice (amys.com).

KIM'S PICK: My son and I are addicted to the No Chicken Noodle
Soup—it's just like traditional chicken noodle, but without the dead
chicken.

Swap that ∿

Campbell's Soup

∿ for this

Progresso Vegetable Classics Soup

Okay, it's not a traditional Skinny Bitch choice, but as a busy mom on
the go, I like to know I have options at my local grocer when I need to
warm them bones. (You can even find Progresso at 7-Eleven!) I find
these soup classics so hearty and filling, but don't go crazy—they're
pretty high in sodium (progressofoods.com).

KIM'S PICKS: My vegan favorites are Lentil, Vegetable Barley,
and Pea.

Muir Glen Organic Soup

I love the way these soups flavor the atmosphere of your whole kitchen.
Try the Savory Lentil and the Southwest Black Bean (muirglen.com).

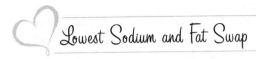
Health Valley Organic Soup

This entire line of canned soups is low in sodium and fat. The soups are a tad bland and don't pack as much flavor, but for the sake of your health (and weight), they're a good indulgence. Try the Lentil, Split Pea, Tomato, Vegetable, Vegetable Barley, Black Bean, or Potato Leek (healthvalley.com).

Ramen Noodles

If you went to college, you know about ramen noodles. You ain't got to lie to kick it, sister. I was broke as a joke and could barely afford a beer, but my dorm room had Top Ramen coming out its ears. I call it Poor Chick's Gourmet. But now if I take a look at the back of the package, I stick my finger in my throat. It's loaded with MSG, sodium, and artificial colors, preservatives, and sugar. Here are a few brands you can swap out for the unhealthy stuff.

Swap that ∿∿∿

Top Ramen

∿∿∿ for this

Dr. McDougall's Baked Ramen Noodles

Cute lil' instant ramen cups filled with baked noodles drowning in a vegetarian broth. They're more noodlelike and less brothy than other ramens, but still have serious flavor despite the lack of MSG. Try Chicken or Beef flavor. For other college dorm favorites, check out the entire line of dry soup cups (rightfoods.com).

Soken Ramen

Gourmet ramen noodles packed in the same scrunchy, plastic bags that are reminiscent of your days as a poor girl. Quick and easy to make, with no preservatives or MSG. Try the Miso Ramen or Brown Rice Ramen (amazon.com).

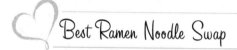

Best Ramen Noodle Swap

Koyo Ramen Noodles

This is another one that's strikingly similar to commercial ramen. The big difference? Koyo's ramen noodles are organic, with all natural ingredients—not the sodium-packed, artificial junk. (Yes, I know, Top Ramen is amazeballs.) You just boil the noodles in water for four minutes, and they expand into a light, brothy soup. The flavor can be a bit bland, so just add some green onions and Braggs Liquid Amino Acids to liven it up. Vegan ramen varieties are available in Seaweed, Mushroom, Tofu and Miso, Asian Vegetable, Garlic Pepper, Soba, and Lemongrass Ginger (koyonaturalfoods.com).

Breads

The bread aisle can be a confusing place, and one that is full of greenwashing. Bread makers know the buzzwords that catch your eye, and they make them as big and as bold as the Hollywood sign whenever they can. Take Wonder Bread, which touts its nutritional value. The only thing I'm left to wonder is how the hell it gets away with it. Glimpse at the back of the label, and you'll find high-fructose corn syrup, mono- and diglycerides (animal fat), sodium stearoyl lactylate (milk product), DATEM (more animal fat), and some sulfates and phosphates. Um, gross.

As a general rule, steer clear of white bread. You want to look for breads that are 100 percent whole grain, meaning the healthy bran and wheat germ haven't been stripped away during processing. Whole-grain breads retain more fiber, protein, vitamins, and minerals, without all the sugar. They make you feel full longer and protect your bangin' body from cardiovascular and gum disease. You won't feel any guilt eating these healthy breads.

Love Force Raw Organic Bread

Slap together two large slices of this all-organic, all-raw energy bread. In my household, we love the Sun-Flax Focaccia made with sunflower seeds, flax seeds, sun-dried tomato, pine nuts, agave nectar, and Italian seasoning; also choose from Sun-Flax Italian, Sun-Flax Raisin, Sun-Flax Original, and Sun-Flax Rye Bread (loveforce.net).

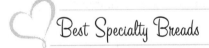 Best Specialty Breads

*Rudi's Organic Bakery

Rudi's is all about using fresh and natural ingredients that you can recognize and pronounce, rather than those that require a freakin' dictionary. Expect just good ole rolled oats, sunflower seeds, oat flour, wheat bran, and barley malt. Available in gluten-free varieties.

Choose from hamburger and hot dog buns in 100% Whole Wheat and in Spelt; 100% Whole Wheat and Artisan Breads in Cinnamon Raisin, Double Fiber, Multigrain Oat, 14 Grain, 7 Grain with Flax, Nut and Oat, Tuscan Roasted Garlic, Rosemary Olive Oil, and European Multigrain (rudisbakery.com).

KIM'S PICK: I absolutely love the Tuscan Roasted Garlic and Rosemary Olive Oil.

Healthiest Breads

*Food for Life Breads

Started in the back of a quaint natural-foods store in Glendale, California, in the 1960s, Food for Life only uses sprouted, certified organic live grains to optimize the nutrients in its breads. I can't get enough of the rich, nutty, crunchy taste. It also makes specialty breads free of gluten, wheat, and yeast for those with allergies. Breads are available in Ezekiel 4:9 Organic Sprouted 100% Whole Grain Flourless Bread and 7 Sprouted Grains Bread; English muffins in Organic Sprouted 100% Whole Grain and Seed, and Wheat and Gluten Free Brown

Sprouting is a good thing. It increases the vitamin content and "predigests" the grains to aid your body in digesting the entire grain.

Rice; and hamburger buns in Ezekiel 4:9 Sprouted Whole Grain Burger Buns (foodforlife.com).

French Meadow Bakery Breads

Whatever type of bread your sandwich calls for, French Meadow's got you covered. Its organic, all-natural breads come in yeast- and gluten-free, sprouted-grain, and kosher and pareve options. Varieties include Hemp Bread (low-glycemic and yeast-free), Healthseed Spelt Bread (organic and yeast-free), and Flax and Sunflower Seed Bread (organic and yeast-free; frenchmeadow.com).

Bagels and English Muffins

Alvarado St. Bakery Breads and Bagels. Located in beautiful Sonoma County, Alvarado Street Bakery produces healthy, certified organic whole-grain breads and bagels with ingredients such as sprouted wheat, unbleached wheat flour, and barley malt. Available in Sprouted Wheat Sesame Bagels, Sprouted Wheat Onion Poppyseed Bagels, and Sprouted Wheat Original Bagels (alvaradostreetbakery.com).

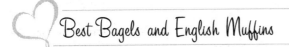
Best Bagels and English Muffins

Rudi's Organic Bakery Bagels and English Muffins

Rudi's has a kick-ass line of kosher organic bagels and English muffins made with the freshest and healthiest ingredients. Plain bagels are available in flavors such as Cinnamon Raisin and Multigrain; English muffins in Multigrain with Flax, Spelt, Whole Grain Wheat, and Harvest Seeded (rudisbakery.com).

KIM'S PICK: Earth Balance up the Multigrain with Flax English muffins and then top with some jam for a special treat.

Orowheat Bagels

I wouldn't give these five stars, because the ingredients aren't anything snazzy, but they are available at major grocery chains and will do in a pinch. Available in Plain, Double Fiber, 100% Whole Wheat, and Cinnamon Raisin (orowheat.com).

Tortillas

Flour and corn tortillas are refined and processed, which strips the grains of all the healthy bran and nutrients. Manufacturers then process them with chemicals and add artificial preservatives to make sure they can hang out on the shelf for a while. Wheat or whole-grain tortillas have a more earthy taste, but they're low-glycemic and better for your bod all around.

*French Meadow Certified Organic Sprouted Grain Tortillas

Yeast- and gluten-free tortillas made by the longest-running USDA-certified organic bakery in the States (frenchmeadow.com).

*Food for Life Tortillas

Making high-quality breads from sprouted grain for more than forty years, Food for Life processes all baking products to ensure they don't lose vital nutrients and natural fibers. No artificial flavors, colors, or preservatives have touched its organic Wheat and Gluten Free Brown Rice Tortillas or Ezekiel 4:9 Sprouted Grain Tortillas (foodforlife.com).

Swap that ∿∿∿↘

↙∿∿∿ *for this*

Indian Life Tortillas

These aren't your mama's tortillas. Make a spicy wrap with these spunky tortillas made from organic flour, spiced vegetables, herbs, and spices. Wraps available in Plain, Spinach, Masala, Coriander, Chapati, Pesto, and Sundried Tomato (indianlife.com).

KIM'S PICK: Pesto Wraps; so soft and fresh, and you can really taste the herbs and spices!

Alvarado St. Bakery Sprouted Wheat Tortillas

Organic whole-wheat flour tortillas made with unrefined safflower oil. Available in Fajita and Burrito sizes (alvaradostreetbakery.com).

Taco Shells

If you need to hear the crunch, then get this: taco shells are typically cooked with partially hydrogenated vegetable oil, which contains trans fat. These jerks increase your bad cholesterol, while decreasing the good. Eating them may also put you at risk of a heart attack or stroke. Any questions?

Bearitos All Natural Taco Shells

Stuff these babies with some lentils and the works, and it's taco time, bitch. Choose from Blue Corn Taco Shells or Yellow Corn Taco Shells, made with organic blue corn and yellow corn flours (littlebear foods.com).

Swap that ∿∿∿

Mission Taco Shells

∿∿∿ *for this*

Garden of Eatin' Taco Shells

Maybe I just like the name, but these certified organic taco shells live up to the hype. Garden of Eatin' also gives you the choice of Yellow Corn Taco Shells or Blue Corn Taco Shells, made with organic stone-ground yellow or blue corn masa flour and safflower and/ or sunflower oils. I love the crispiness of the Blue Corn Taco Shells (gardenofeatin.com).

Croutons

You can tear that aisle apart like a madwoman, but almost every crouton brand you'll find now contains dairy and eggs. For those of us who still appreciate a crunchy treat without robbing a cow, here are a few gourmet vegan varieties with no yucky chemicals or preservatives.

Edward & Sons Organic Croutons

Add some zesty flavor to soups or salads with organic croutons made from whole-grain wheat and seasonings. Available in Italian Herbs and Onion Garlic (edwardandsons.com).

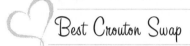

Best Crouton Swap

Melissa's Good Life Food Organic Croutons

One hundred percent organic croutons with no MSG. Not all of the varieties are vegan, but look for the Garden Herb and the Tomato and Basil (melissas.com).

Chips and Crackers

To prevent myself from making a run to the border—Taco Bell, that is—I need to pack my pantry and purse with good, healthy snacks. Chips and crackers fill the void when you feel like you're headed for a junk-food binge, and if you pick the right ones, they are chock-full of fiber and nutrients. Here are a few snack brands that work to eliminate the icky ingredients, but remember, everything in moderation.

Chips

Trader Joe's Potato Chips

This is your chip, bitch. Let the truth be told: once you pop one, you really can't stop with Trader Joe's signature potato and tortilla chips.

Most are lower in saturated fat and higher in omega-3s and fiber, so you can shed a little guilt. Try the Trio Unsalted Thick Cut Red Bliss, Blue and Yukon Gold Potato Chips, Kettle Cooked Olive Oil Potato Chips (only 0.5 grams of saturated fat), Trader Joe's Popped Potato Chips Salted (a popular choice), Organic Blue Corn Tortilla Chips, White Corn Tortilla Chips Unsalted, and Soy and Flaxseed Tortilla Chips (traderjoes.com).

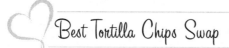

Best Tortilla Chips Swap

Trader Joe's Veggie and Flaxseed Tortilla Chips

These übercolorful veggie and flaxseed tortilla chips have a slight nuttiness and a savory deliciousness thanks to carrots, tomato, spinach, garlic, red beets, and onion. They are perfect for dipping in guacamole or salsa (traderjoes.com).

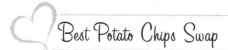

Best Potato Chips Swap

Kettle Brand Potato Chips

Kettle cooks its potatoes in the finest oils and then lightly seasons them with natural ingredients and spices for a fresh yet flavored-packed crunch. They have a certain crunchiness to them that other chips don't. Vegan varieties available in Salt and Fresh Ground Pepper, and Sea Salt and Vinegar (kettlebrand.com).

Swap that ⌒⌒⌒⌒⌒

Cheese puffs

⌒⌒⌒⌒⌒ for this

*Pirate's Booty Puffs, Veggie

With 50 percent less fat than regular potato chips and all-natural ingredients, Pirate's Booty vegan-friendly puffs are made from puffed rice and corn and a medley of vegetables such as spinach, kale, carrots, and parsley. Thankfully, the veggies don't overpower the cheesy corn flavor. They are smaller than typical cheese puffs, but all the better—you can shovel a handful into your mouth all at once (pirate brands.com).

Swap that ⌒⌒⌒⌒⌒

Frito-Lay Cheetos

⌒⌒⌒⌒⌒ for this

*Original Tings Crunchy Corn Sticks

Step away from the Cheetos. Are you asking for trouble? Pirate Brands' Original Tings are to die for, and so much better for you than the toxic cheesy puffs. But they are no less addictive. You still get the rich, cheesy flavor, but they are so light and crunchy (piratebrands.com).

*Potato Flyers Homestyle Barbeque

Another winner from Pirate's Brands, Potato Flyers are baked with a special combo of tomatoes, spices, and a sweet, smoky BBQ flavor (piratebrands.com).

Crackers

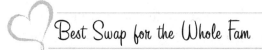

Best Swap for the Whole Fam

Late July Organic Crackers, Peanut Butter

Bite-size sandwich crackers made with real organic peanut butter. The small, family-owned company also makes a line of organic multi-grain chips (gluten-free) that will drive you nuts (latejuly.com).

Swap that ○○○○○

Nabisco Triscuits

○○○○○ for this

Back to Nature's Harvest Whole Wheat Crackers

Made from 100 percent whole grain, Back to Nature's Harvest Whole Wheat Crackers are similar to Triscuits, but without the fake flavors, preservatives, and food dyes. They are a dead ringer for the commercial brand, but they have real, natural homemade flavor (backto naturefoods.com).

fat
fact

Potato chips were created to piss some-one off. Well, sort of. A chef named George Strum was trying to get back at some jerk who complained that his French fries were too thick. Way to show him.

Swap that ⟶

for this

Back to Nature's Crispy Wheat Crackers

If you're more of a Wheat Thin type, these crispy wheat crackers have your name written all over 'em. A perfect hearty snack with Daiya cheese or vegan pâté (backtonaturefoods.com).

Swap that ⟶

Cheez-It Crackers

for this

Eco-Planet Non-Dairy Cheddar Crackers

These taste just like the Cheez-Its I used to love growing up. Plus, they're shaped like mini suns, earths, wind machines, and electric cars to get you thinking about clean energy (ecoheavenllc.com).

*Myrna's Skinny Crisps

These low-carb, gluten-free crackers, made from organic ground flax-seeds, almonds, and chickpea flour, are baked to perfection. Available in Toasty Onion, Plain Jane, White Sesame Seed, Cinnamon, and Chocolate Brownie (skinnycrisps.com).

Popcorn

Enough with the microwave popcorn already. Did you know you're breathing in dozens of chemicals every time you open a piping hot bag? From the ingredients that impart the buttery flavor to the inks and glues on the bag, some of these chemicals turn toxic when heated to high temperatures (say, like in a microwave . . .). And guess who's breathing in that extra buttery aroma? Yes, that would be you, babe.

There's more bad news. Orville Redenbacher, the godfather of the popcorn industry, thinks it's cute to market his microwave popcorn as a "healthful snack." Close, but no cigar. Just one serving contains 30 percent of your daily recommended value of saturated fat. That's not the stuff you should be sneaking into the movie theater. (Oh, don't act like you're above that.) Instead, pop some of these kernels into your mouth next time you're jonesing for a movie snack.

*Popcorn, Indiana All Natural Kettlecorn

Gluten-free with no saturated fat, Popcorn, Indiana uses pure cane sugar and the finest whole grains for their signature kettlecorn. Vegan varieties are available in Cinnamon Sugar, Cocoa Kettle, and Original Kettlecorn. If you really want to send your taste buds into overdrive, try the Reserve Popcorn in Wasabi (popcornindiana.com).

NOW Foods Certified Organic Popcorn Kernels

Yes, believe it or not, people used to actually make it on the stove . . . not in the microwave. Ditch the phony microwave garbage, and make your popcorn on the stove with these kernels. Enjoy a movie with the same soft puffs that melt on your tongue without the additives and pesticides (nowfoods.com).

Popcorn Toppings

Popcorn can be so mundane. Liven things up by adding fun toppings such as Spanish smoked paprika, nutritional yeast, cayenne powder, chili pepper, curry powder, cumin, grated vegan parmesan cheese, or sriracha (a Thai hot sauce).

Swap that

Orville Redenbacher's Gourmet Popping Corn

for this

Eden Organic Popping Corn

Eden takes extra care to make sure the corn kernels retain moisture and aren't scratched or damaged in transit from the farm to the packaging plant. Popcorn that's treated like fine diamonds—just my style (edenfoods.com).

177

Stovetop Popcorn

Yield: 2 quarts

3 tablespoons peanut or grapeseed oil
⅓ cup kernels
1 (3-quart) covered saucepan
2 tablespoons Earth Balance nondairy butter, or more to taste

Heat the oil in the saucepan on medium-high heat. Put 3 or 4 popcorn kernels into the oil and cover the pan. When the kernels pop, add the remainder of the popcorn kernels in an even layer. Cover, remove from heat, and count for 30 seconds. (There's a reason for all this. You are first heating the oil; then by waiting 30 seconds, you give the other kernels a chance to near popping temperature, so that when you set them back on heat, they all pop at about the same time.)

Return the pan to the heat. The popcorn should begin popping soon, all at once. Once the popping starts, gently shake the pan by moving it back and forth over the burner. Try to keep the lid slightly ajar to let the steam from the popcorn release. Once the popping slows to several seconds between pops, remove the pan from the heat, remove the lid, and dump the popcorn immediately into a wide bowl. (With this technique, almost all of the kernels pop and nothing burns.)

If you are adding Earth Balance, you can easily melt it by placing the butter in the now empty, but hot pan. Salt to taste.

Quick Tip: If you add salt to the oil in the pan before popping, the salt will distribute throughout the pan as the popcorn pops.

Cereal

Quit digging through the box for that little prize. Are you five? The only treasure you're going to find is a heap of sugar. Not really the temporary tattoo you were hoping for, huh? Although most cereals claim to trim your waistline and be good for your heart, they don't deserve the healthy image. It's called advertising. And you fell for it. How much sugar we talking about? The equivalent of three large spoonfuls per serving. Of the cereals targeted at kiddies, nine out of ten are loaded in sugar. Breakfast of champions, my ass.

Cold Cereal

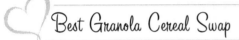

Best Granola Cereal Swap

Trader Joe's Granola Cereal

Fill up on fiber, vitamins, and nutrients with Trader Joe's crunchy bits of baked granola. Available in Lowfat Granola Cereal with Almonds, Organic Granny's Apple Granola Cereal, Organic Mango Passion Granola Cereal (fan-freakin-tastic!), and Oat n' Wheat Bran Swirls (traderjoes.com).

*Barbara's Cereals

Chow down on a bowl of natural, wholesome ingredients, including whole oats and wheat grains, flax, cranberry, and cocoa. Available in Shredded Spoonfuls Multigrain, Puffins Multigrain, Puffins Cinnamon, Puffins Original, and Puffins Peanut Butter (barbarasbakery.com).

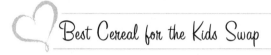

*Nature's Path Envirokidz Organic Cereal

If you have any rug rats in the house, this cereal not only appeals to kids; it's also good for them. Gluten-free and low in sugar. Available in Gorilla Munch Cereal and Peanut Butter Panda Puffs (natures path.com).

Swear Off Those Sugary Cereals

Drop the zero and get with a hero. These healthy cereals taste just like the real thang, but don't come with the artificial dyes, preservatives, and added sugar.

Swap that: **Kellogg's Frosted Flakes**
   for this: **Trader Joe's Frosted Flakes**
Packs the same crunchy, sweet corn flavor, but much healthier (traderjoes.com).

Swap that: **General Mills' Cheerios**
   for this: **Trader Joe's O's Toasted Whole Grain Oats**
Wholesome little o's made from whole-grain oats
(also comes in Sweet Honey Nut; traderjoes.com).

Swap that: **Nabisco Shredded Wheat**
   for this: **Kashi's Autumn Wheat**
So similar to the real thing, you won't know the difference (kashi.com).

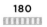

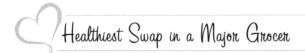

Kashi Cold Cereals

Kashi's certified organic cereals are low in fat and filling, to start your morning off right. Tempt your sweet tooth with Strawberry Fields, filled with crispy rice and organic strawberries and raspberries. Be careful not to eat the bowl (kashi.com).

Swap that: **Kellogg's Frosted Mini-Wheats**
for this: **Arrowhead Mills Shredded Wheat**
Made with high-fiber, organic whole wheat, these bite-size pieces of shredded wheat come in sweetened and unsweetened (arrowheadmills.com).

Swap that: **Kellogg's Fruit Loops**
for this: **Cascadian Farm Organic Fruitful O's**
Go ahead and let the kids chow down on these chunky, fruit-flavored loops—they come without the artificial dyes and preservatives (cascadianfarm.com).

Swap that: **Kellogg's Cinnamon Toast Crunch**
for this: **Cascadian Farm Organic Cinnamon Crunch**
Thin, heavenly organic whole-grain squares dipped in cinnamon and sugar. Yummy for breakfast or as a snack (cascadianfarm.com).

Arrowhead Mills Cold Cereals

Whether you like granola, flakes, or shredded wheat, Arrowhead Mills has a fab selection of all-natural cereals. Flakes are available in Spelt, Oat Bran, Kamut, and Amaranth Multi-grain. Breadshop Granola comes in Crunchy Oat Bran with Almonds and Raisins, Mocha Almond Crunch, Strawberry 'n' Cream, and Raspberry 'n' Cream. The whole-grain puff cereals take the cake, with a yummy, light crunch; available in Wheat, Rice, Millet, Kamut, and Corn (arrowheadmills.com).

Back to Nature Granolas

Sweetened with fruit and cane juices, these whole-grain granolas are straight from nature. Vegan varieties include Apple Blueberry, Classic, Blueberry Walnut, and Chocolate Delight (backtonaturefoods.com).

Cascadian Farm Organic Kids' Cereals

Organic cereals nurtured on a twenty-eight-acre farm in western Washington's North Cascades mountains. Some of our family favorites are the Clifford Crunch, Organic Raisin Bran, and Multigrain Squares (cascadianfarm.com).

Oatmeal

Best On-the-Go Oatmeal Swap

*Dr. McDougall's Organic Cereal Big Cups

Hearty, multigrain hot cereals in cute little cups. Available in Peach Raspberry with Organic Grains, Cranberry Muesli with Organic Grains, Organic Maple 4-Grain with Real Maple, and Organic Apple Cinnamon Oatmeal and Wheat (rightfoods.com).

Trader Joe's Quick Cook Steel Cut Oats

Steel-cut oats have a reputation for taking a long time to make, but these cook quickly and have a nuttier flavor than oatmeal (traderjoes.com).

Country Choice Organic Canister Hot Cereals

Certified organic hot cereals in Irish Style Steel Cut Oats and Multigrain Hot Cereal (countrychoiceorganic.com).

Most Original Swap

McCann's Imported Irish Oatmeal

The brand behind the famous steel-cut Irish oatmeal, these 100 percent whole-grain Irish oats have a hearty, nutty flavor and are oh-so-filling. McCann's oatmeals come in 28-ounce tins with nothing artificial. Available in Steel-Cut Irish Oatmeal, Quick and Easy Steel-

Cut Irish Oatmeal, Quick Cooking Irish Oatmeal, and Instant Irish Oatmeal (mccanns.ie).

Instant Oatmeal

Trader Joe's Instant Oatmeal

Warm up with a pipin' hot bowl of whole-grain oatmeal pumped with fiber, vitamins, and minerals. Available in Maple and Brown Sugar, Organic Oats and Flax, and Organic Cinnamon Spice (trader joes.com).

*Arrowhead Mills Hot Cereals

Quick and easy-to-prepare organic grains. Available in Organic Steel Cut Oats, Instant Oatmeal Original Plain, Instant Organic Oatmeal with Flax, Organic Oat Bran, and Instant Oatmeal Maple Apple Spice. You fickle bitches should try the Instant Organic Oatmeal Variety Pack with three different flavors (arrowheadmills.com).

Best Instant Oatmeal Swap

Nature's Path Instant Hot Oatmeal

Ready in minutes, these oatmeal packets are hearty and healthy, with dried fruit and nuts. The Maple Nut is a must try. Available in nine flavors, including Maple Nut, Apple Cinnamon, Multigrain Raisin Spice, Flax Plus with Omega-3s, and Hemp Plus with Omega-3s (naturespath.com).

Available in Organic Steel-Cut Oats and Organic Rolled Oats (king arthurflour.com).

Mac 'n' Cheese

No, you're not going nuckin' futs. It's vegan mac 'n' cheese in a box! I wasn't always a big fan of the traditional version, but it's great to have on hand to shut the kids up.

$Swap\ that$ ᘣᘣᘣᘣ

Kraft Macaroni and Cheese

ᘣᘣᘣᘣ $for\ this$

Road's End Organics Mac and Chreese

Not one, but five mac 'n' cheese flavors that are free of dairy, soy, and cholesterol. It's not the best stuff on the shelf, but if you're a mac 'n' cheese fanatic and need an alternative, it fits the bill. It has a lighter cheesy flavor than Kraft, so it doesn't feel so heavy on the tummy. Try the Shells and Chreese Cheddar Style, Mac and Chreese Alfredo Style (gluten-free), Penne and Chreese Cheddar Style, and 123'z and Chreese Cheddar Style "4 Kidz" (edwardandsons.com).

Leahey Gardens Macaroni and Cheese

Elbow macaroni in a creamy cheeselike sauce (leaheyfoods.com).

Instant Mashed Potatoes

Mashed potatoes are easy to prepare, and they make a great hearty side for dinner. The problem is most boxed brands are crammed with crap. Some brands brag that their mashed potatoes are made with 100 percent real mashed potatoes . . . huh? WTF does that mean? Here's what else they're made with—corn syrup, MSG, partially hydrogenated oils, artificial flavors and dyes, buttermilk, and more milk. First off, milk is a no-no. Duh. And you would be smart to keep the rest of the ingredients off your plate too (not to mention your kids' plates, honey).

*Edward & Sons Mashed Potatoes

These organic mashed potatoes in a box have the same consistency and fluffiness you're used to, but with healthy, gluten-free ingredients. Plus, they're easy to prepare if you're in a rush. Try the Home Style Organic Mashed Potatoes, Roasted Garlic Organic Mashed Potatoes, and Dairy Free Chreesy Organic Mashed Potatoes (edwardandsons.com).

Nutrition Bars

We've all been there. You just finished working out at the gym and all of the sudden you start to feel like ass. Your blood sugar is crashing, and you're tired, bitchy, and just want to rob a 7-Eleven for all the Flamin' Hot Cheetos and Twix bars they have in stock. Chill out, honey. Instead of reaching for junk, keep a good stash of nutrition bars on hand in your purse and car for a healthy, satisfying snack. Not a Power Bar. Instead look for bars that will provide an instant pick-me-up with fruit sweeteners, and nuts and seeds for protein and fiber.

Cereal Bars

*Glutino Gluten Free Breakfast Bars

For breakfast on the go, try these vegan nutritional bars in Strawberry, Apple, Blueberry, and Cherry (glutino.com).

Best Cereal Bar Swap

Barbara's Nature's Choice Multigrain Cereal Bars

Healthy and filling bars wrapped in whole grains like oats and barley and sweetened only with fruit. These bars should be a staple in every pantry. Available in Triple Berry, Apple Cinnamon, Strawberry, Raspberry, Cherry, and Blueberry (barbarasbakery.com).

*Enjoy Life Chewy On-the-Go Bars

Fortified with essential vitamins and minerals, these snack bars are awesome for breakfast or a midday snack. Plus, every bar is free of gluten, dairy, peanuts, tree nuts, soy, and eggs. Available in Very Berry, Cocoa Loco, Sunbutter Crunch (no nuts), and Caramel Apple (enjoylifefoods.com).

Protein and Energy Bars

Vega Whole Food Energy Bars

These are made entirely with plant-based ingredients such as hemp protein, organic sprouted flaxseeds, and organic wheatgrass. For a boost any time of the day, they are an awesome source of protein, fiber, enzymes, phytonutrients, and omega-3 and omega-6 essential fatty acids. Called Vegan Whole Food Vibrancy Bars, available in Chocolate Decadence, Green Synergy, and Wholesome Original (myvega.com).

*Greens Plus 22 Days Energy Bars

Because it takes twenty-one days to break bad habits, Greens Plus developed these energy bars to help you make it to twenty-two. Derived from raw and organic superfoods, they are gluten-free, with plenty of vitamins, minerals, and antioxidants. Available in Cherry Chocolate, Daily Mocha Mantra, Enlightened Pumpkinseed, and Nut Butter Buddha (greensplus.com).

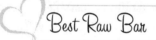 Best Raw Bar

*Pure Bars

I go gaga for these gluten-free bars. They have an unbelievable taste and chunky texture and come in plenty of flavors, so you never get tired of eating them. Pure Naturals are available in Chocolate Almond, Peanut Raisin Crunch, and Superfruit Nutty Crunch; Pure Organic, in Chocolate Brownie, Wild Blueberry, Cherry Cashew, Apple Cinnamon, and Cranberry Orange (thepurebar.com).

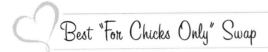

Best "For Chicks Only" Swap

Luna Bars

Designed for chicks by chicks, Luna Bars provide whole nutrition to promote breast health, a balanced diet, and optimal fitness. Although the bars are organic, they contain a bit too many ingredients for my liking. Still they are supereasy to find and taste like a crunchy, crispy cookie. A pointer: they don't contain dairy, but the package says that may contain traces of dairy (probably because of the facility they're made in). If you are seriously a hard-core vegan, this may not be the bar for you. But if a little trace doesn't get your panties in a bunch, then go for it. Connect four, sister. Widely available at major grocers and natural-food stores in Chocolate Peppermint Stick, Dulce de Leche, S'mores, and White Chocolate Macadamia (lunabar.com).

Swap that ᛣᛣᛣᛣᛣ

Nature Valley Granola Bars

ᛣᛣᛣᛣᛣ for this

*Lärabars

Deelish fruit and nut bars packin' only a few ingredients—all of which you can find in your pantry. No artificial coloring, additives, and preservatives. They are soft, chewy, fruity, low in carbs and so insanely good. My personal favorite? Cherry Pie. Also available in Blueberry Muffin, Coconut Cream Pie, and Key Lime Pie (larabar.com).

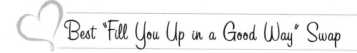
Best "Fill You Up in a Good Way" Swap

*MacroBars

Get a nice, natural rush with these pure vegan, macrobiotic bars that use the simplest of ingredients to boost your immunity and give you essential nutrients. I was initially put off by the fact that they are macrobiotic, but they're moist and wildly fruity with a mild oat flavor. No additives, preservatives, refined sugars or flours, so your bod stays balanced. Available in Chocolate Crunch, Cashew Butter, Granola with Coconut, Peanut Butter Chocolate Chip, Banana Almond, Almond Butter with Carob, Tahini Date, and Cashew Caramel (gomacro.com).

*Sun Flour Baking California Bar

Inspired by the active California lifestyle, this bar is packed with raisins, walnuts, flaxseeds, chocolate chips, and rice crisp. A great tasting gluten-free snack that even your kids will scribble on the grocery list (sunflourbaking.com).

Baked Goods

*Amy's Organic Cakes

Irresistible, boxed organic pound cakes made with cocoa powder, apple cider vinegar, vanilla extract, and evaporated cane juice. Vegan varieties available in Chocolate, Chocolate Gluten Free, and Orange (amys.com).

Glenny's Brown Rice Marshmallow Treats

Whole-grain brown rice mixed with wholesome, organic marshmallow ingredients and pressed into ricey cakes. Low in calories and gluten-free. Available in Chocolate, Peanut Caramel, Raspberry Jubilee, and Vanilla (glennys.com).

Swap that ∿∿∿∿↘

Hostess Twinkies

↙∿∿∿∿ *for this*

X's to O's Vegan Bakery Canoe Boats

No, these aren't going to make you skinny, but they are oh-so-sweet. (Remember I'm not here to judge, just make referrals.) The signature Canoe Boats—spongy cakes stuffed with a cream filling—look just like Twinkies, but are plumper. Available in Chocolate Covered, Vanilla, Cookies and Cream, Carrot Cake, and Strawberries and Cream. Shop online and have them shipped to your doorstep (xoxovegan bakery.com).

Swap that ⟋⟋⟋⟋⟍

Hostess Ding Dongs

⟋⟋⟋⟋⟍ *for this*

Moo-Cluck Crème-Filled Cupcakes

Made fresh and shipped frozen (shop online), Moo-Cluck's cupcakes are all vegan, all made with nonhydrogenated oils, and all injected with a creamy filling. My favorite are the Chocolate Cupcakes filled with vanilla or peanut butter cream and topped with chocolate ganache (moocluck.com).

⟶ *The perfect treat when you're PMSing! A good vice to keep you from ripping everyone's head off.*

Doughnuts

Swap that ⟋⟋⟋⟋⟍

Dunkin' Donuts Munchkins

⟋⟋⟋⟋⟍ *for this*

Nutrilicious Donut Holes

These satisfied my Dunkin' Donuts pregnancy cravings. Made with natural ingredients and no artificial colors, flavors, or hydrogenated oils.

Available in Carrot Cake, Chocolate Carob Glazed, Soy Yogurt Glazed, Gingerbread, Pumpkin, and Blueberry (store.veganessentials.com).

VeganSweets Donuts

Chocolate or vanilla donuts specially made with ingredients such as wheat flour, evaporated cane juice, and fruit juice. Each one is topped with frosting. Heat them up for an extra messy treat (veganstore.com).

Blondies

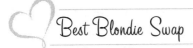

Best Blondie Swap

*Sun Flour Baking Blondies

Soft, buttery bars with a rich butterscotch flavor. The molasses gives them a sensational chewy texture (sunflourbaking.com).

Frankly Natural Bakers Vegan Decadence Blondies

So rich, so wickedly sweet, and so without the eggs and dairy that make up a traditional blondie. These are made with organic oat flour and only pure, natural ingredients (no wheat). Available in Chocolate, Butterscotch, and Café Latte (franklynatural.com).

Brownies

Swap that ⟳⟳⟳⟳⟳↘

Little Debbie Fudge Brownies

↙⟲⟲⟲⟲⟲ for this

Allison's Gourmet Vegan Brownies

To hell with Little Debbie. These brownies look and taste like they're straight out of Martha's pantry. Made with 100 percent organic ingredients and fair-trade chocolate, they're amazingly moist and sweet. Try the Pecan Brownie, which has all the nuts and brownie goodness you'll ever need. Also available in Original, Double Chocolate, Brazil Nut, Cherry Chocolate, Amaretto Almond, and Half Original/Half Pecan (allisonsgourmet.com).

*Sun Flour Baking Brownie Bears

I'm a sucker for brownies, and it's tough to find a scrumptious one that isn't made with eggs and dairy. These are not only vegan, but also gluten-free and free of hydrogenated oils (sunflourbaking.com).

Candy

Something tells me I don't need to sell you on why candy is bad for you. Call it a hunch. It's not such a bad thing to indulge in a Twix on a road trip or Snickers to satisfy a craving on occasion, but I think we can all agree on this: if it's in your house, you're gonna eat it, woman. Keep telling yourself it's there for emergencies. But last time I checked, your sweet tooth is not the best judge of what's considered an emergency. Am I right, or am I right? You won't feel like such a bloated mess if you swap out for the confections below. That still doesn't mean you can buy all the stock in the store. It's still candy, and you still have no self-control.

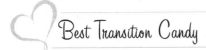

Best Transition Candy

*The Ginger People Ginger Chews

Individually wrapped, chewy candies with a spicy ginger kick. My son refers to them as the "spicy candy" whenever he wants me to dig one out of my purse. I love these with a passion, and they just happen to help with motion and morning sickness, thanks to the powerful effects of ginger. Available in Original, Peanut Ginger, and Spicy Apple (gingerpeople.com).

Swap that ✎

Chupa Chups Lollipops

✎ for this

*YummyEarth Organic Lollipops

Here's how this is going to work. You're going to buy these for your kid. Then your kid is going to hand you a leftover pop when he's got something better to do. Then you're going to finish it because that's what moms do. Then you're going to hide the rest of the bag from your kid, because the temptation to rip one out of his mouth while he's happily enjoying it will be far too great for a mother to bear. Got it?

These lollipops come in twenty-one tantalizing, gluten-free flavors with all-organic ingredients and real fruit extract, including Wet-Face Watermelon, TooBerry Blueberry, Googly Grape, Very Very Cherry, Sour Apple Tart, Pomegranate Pucker, Mango Tango, Roadside Root Beer, Hopscotch Butterscotch, and Strawberry Smash (yummyearth.com).

Swap that ⁓⁓⁓⁓

Haribo Gold-Bears Gummi Candy

⁓⁓⁓ *for this*

*Surf Sweets Organic and Natural Candy

Just what the dentist ordered—the best gummy knockoffs on the market, sweetened with organic fruit juice and colors from nature. I'm not one to tout the health benefits of candy, but just one serving earns you 100 percent of your recommended daily value of vitamin C. Vegan candies available in Gummy Swirls, Fruity Bears, Sour Worms, and Sour Berry Bears (just like Sour Patch Kids; surfsweets.com).

Swap that ~~~

~~~ for this

*Candy Tree Organic Candy Licorice

Finally, something better to sneak into the movie theater! Get over your Red Vines and Twizzlers fascination—seriously, the list of ingredients is two miles long in those, honey! These are still chewy and fruity, and so much better for you than the crap behind the theater snack bar. Candy Tree's licorice vines and twists are made with organic ingredients, concentrated fruit juice, and carnauba wax. Much better. Available in Licorice Twists, Cherry Twists, Licorice Laces, Raspberry Laces, and Strawberry Laces (naturalwebstore.com).

Chocolate

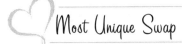 Most Unique Swap

Ecco Bella Health by Chocolate

If Victoria's Secret made chocolate, this would be the push-up bra. Truth be told, I'm not a big fan of dark chocolate, but these organic dark chocolate bars are so light and smooth—without the bitter taste. Each one is fortified with herbs, antioxidants, vitamins, and minerals

fat fact

Ever wonder why chocolate makes people all lovey dovey? It contains a natural substance called phenylethylamine (PEA), which is believed to activate the same feeling in the body as when you're falling for someone.

for all your womanly needs. Available in Beautiful Bones (boosts bone mass and density), Women's Wonder (helps support balanced hormone levels), and Instant Bliss Beauty (corrects skin imbalances . . . hello, zits?! healthbychocolate.com).

KIM'S PICK: I'm slightly obsessed with the Women's Wonder, because it contains rose oil, an intense flavor that pops through in each bite.

Best Damn Dark Chocolate Bar Swap

Endangered Species Organic Dark Chocolate Bars

This boutique chocolate maker offers a nice variety of dark chocolate flavors that don't have that bitter taste. Three-ounce bars are available in plain or with additions like Cacao Nibs, Yacon, and Acai; Goji Berry, Pecans, and Maca; and Golden Berry and Lucuma (chocolatebar.com).

KIM'S PICK: Bite down on the Organic Dark Chocolate with Goji Berry, Pecans, and Maca—my ultimate vice.

I'm all for satisfying my premenstrual needs with a fat bar of chocolate—especially when that chocolate gives back. Every year, Endangered Species Chocolate donates 10 percent of profits to organizations that support species and habitat conservation efforts.

Conscious Creations Dark Chocolate Covered Hazelnuts

There's a reason they call this the "Food of the Goddess." Because only a goddess adds protein to her diet with roasted hazelnuts smothered in certified organic dark chocolate. Conscious Creations uses Rapadura brand unrefined organic sugar in place of processed sugars, so you get a healthy rush (store.veganessentials.com).

Chocolove Premium Belgian Chocolate Bars

Been a while since anybody sexed you up? Make yourself feel wanted with a sensual blend of cocoa and exotic herbs, dried fruits, and nuts. Each bar is presented like a love letter, complete with romantic poems inside each wrapper. The vegan dark chocolate bars are available with such wonderful additions as Cherries and Almonds, Raspberries, Almonds and Sea Salt, Orange Peel, Crystallized Ginger, Chilies and Cherries, and Peppermint (chocolove.com).

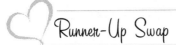 Runner-Up Swap

Newman's Own Organics Signature Series Chocolate

For all you do-gooders, Newman's flavorful dark chocolate is made from certified organic cocoa beans grown on Rainforest Alliance Certified farms. Each bar has a slight sweetness that balances the strong dark chocolate taste. Vegan chocolate available in Dark, Super Dark, Espresso Dark, and Orange Dark (newmansownorganics.com).

KIM'S PICK: Orange Dark Chocolate.

Chocolate Decadence Bars

Listen up, Willy Wonka. This is how chocolate is done. With one of the best varieties of dairy- and gluten-free chocolate, Chocolate Decadence hand-pours and hand-dips all of its chocolate-covered bars, trail mixes, pretzels, and nuts. Choose from bars in Chocolate Almond, Mint Chocolate, Dark Chocolate, Pure Dark Chocolate, and Chocolate Pretzel (chocolatedecadence.com).

*Cocomels Chocolate Covered Coconut Milk Caramels

Sweet, vegan caramels wrapped in dark vegan chocolate and sweetened with brown rice syrup and evaporated cane juice. Gluten- and soy-free. Choose from chocolates in plain, Chai, Fleur de Sel (Sea Salt), or Vanilla, or get all four with the sampler (store.veganessentials.com).

Swap that 〜〜〜〜

Reese's Peanut Butter Cups

〜〜〜 for this

Justin's Nut Butter Organic Dark Chocolate Peanut Butter Cups

Trade in the Reese's Peanut Butter Cups for these doppelgangers. These peanut butter cups contain all organic ingredients such as dark chocolate, evaporated cane sugar, chocolate liquor, cocoa butter, soy lecithin, vanilla, peanut butter, and dry roasted nuts. Reese's on the other hand . . . not so much (justinsnutbutter.com).

Frozen Food Swaps

Waffles

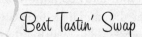 Best Tastin' Swap

*Nature's Path Organic Waffles

Nutritious frozen waffles that are crispy, yet mouthwateringly soft. They are made with organic ingredients and natural grains and seeds such as quinoa, flax, hemp, and buckwheat. Great for breakfast or as a midday snack. Gluten-free flavors available (naturespath.com).

An asterisk (*) means the product is gluten-free.

KIM'S PICK: The Buckwheat Wildberry has a sweet berry flavor, but isn't overpowering.

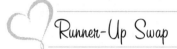 *Runner-Up Swap*

Van's Waffles

Van's makes fluffy and flavorful waffles in Wheat Free/Gluten Free and Organic. The line is easier to find in traditional grocers and offers a nice variety of flavors. Wheat Free/Gluten Free is available in Totally Natural, Blueberry, Apple Cinnamon, Buckwheat, Minis, and Flax; Organic, in Blueberry, Flax, and Totally Natural (vansfoods.com).

Burritos

Cheap, easy, and hot in minutes. No, I'm not talking about your college days, you sleaze. I'm talking about the loathsome frozen burrito. Just one burrito delivers an average of 25 percent of your daily sodium intake, 21 percent of your recommended total fat for the day, and little to nothing in the vitamins and minerals department. Here are some healthier burritos to stuff in your freezer while you're going through the "change."

Evol Classic Burrito, Veggie Fajita

Assorted bell peppers, black beans, and brown rice topped with a tomato and roasted corn salsa in a whole-wheat flour tortilla. Made with 70 percent organic ingredients (evolfoods.com).

Evol Classic Burrito, Tofu and Spinach Sauté

Roasted potatoes, black beans, and sautéed spinach and tofu topped with a tomato and roasted corn salsa in a whole-wheat flour tortilla. Made with 80 percent organic ingredients (evolfoods.com).

*Amy's Black Bean Vegetable Burrito

Organic black beans and veggies nestled in an organic flour tortilla. Spicy just the way I like it (amys.com).

*Amy's Indian Spinach Tofu Wrap

Organic spinach, onions, garlic, ginger, and tofu wrapped in a whole-wheat tortilla (amys.com).

*Amy's Gluten-Free Non-Dairy Burrito

Organic rice, pinto beans, and veggies in a light Mexican sauce, rolled up in a gluten-free tortilla (amys.com).

Moo Moo's Chipotle Black Bean Burrito

My version of "the works," this sensational burrito is a spinach tortilla stuffed with smoked chipotle black beans, Southwest tofu strips, roasted bell peppers, and avocado smothered in a roasted corn salsa (moomooscuisine.com).

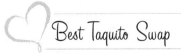 Best Taquito Swap

*Starlite Cuisine's Soy Taquitos and Crispy Rolled Tacos

GMO-free, soy "meat" taquitos and tacos hand-rolled in corn or flour tortillas. Tons of spices perk up these babies. Taquitos available in Original Beef Style, Meatless Chicken Style, and Soy Chorizo and Black Bean Style. Tacos available in Chipotle Chicken Style, Garlic Chicken Style, and Santa Fe Chicken Style (starlitecuisine.com).

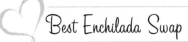 Best Enchilada Swap

Trader Joe's Black Bean and Corn Enchiladas

These are living proof that enchiladas don't need cheese to make you swoon. Covered in a rich black bean sauce, they are a tad on the spicy side. Take them to work and pop in the microwave for a quick, but not too filling lunch (traderjoes.com).

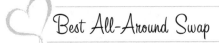 Best All-Around Swap

*Amy's Bean and Rice Burrito

Just tasty rice and beans wrapped in a classic soft, flavorful tortilla. So simple, yet so satisfying (amys.com).

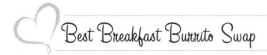

*Amy's Breakfast Burrito

This should be illegal for breakfast. Laugh all you want, but once you bite down on this organic flour wrap filled with organic potatoes, tofu, black beans, veggies, and salsa, you'll look guilty (amys.com).

A Bitch I Love

Tamale Molly

Erin Wood brings a whole new meaning to the term "conscious eater." After years of training stockbrokers, she decided she would take the skills her mama gave her and give back to the hungry. That's how Erin went from being a numbers cruncher to leading a small team of eight who hand-tie more than forty-five hundred tamales a day. If her vegan tamales (in the spirit of transparency, she makes meat versions too), made with extra virgin olive oil and fresh ingredients and tied in a natural corn husk, don't paint a halo over her head, then her charity will—Erin donates every dime of profit to local food banks.

Available in Vegan Red Chili with Peppers and Olives, Vegan Chard and Shallots, and Vegan Black Bean with Chipotle Chile. Find them at Whole Foods Market or online at amazon.com.

*Amy's Light in Sodium Bean and Rice Burrito

Basically the Bean and Rice Burrito, but with half the sodium (amys.com).

Lightlife Smart Tortilla Wrap, Ranchero

Low in fat and sodium, this wrap packs chick'n "veggie" strips, brown rice, and veggies in a mild cilantro sauce (lightlife.com).

Breakfast Meals

Amy's Tofu Scramble

A filling, organic tofu scramble with assorted veggies and hash browned taters. Tastes like a home-cooked meal, but with little effort (amys.com).

*Amy's Black Bean Tamale Verde

Maybe not your traditional breakfast, but you're not a traditional broad, are you? Keep things interesting with organic black beans, chilis, jalapenos, and a handful of fresh vegetables wrapped in organic masa. After the whole shebang is folded and steamed, the tamale is unwrapped, topped with verde sauce, and, just to make sure you're stuffed, accompanied by a side of Spanish brown rice (amys.com).

*Amy's Breakfast Burrito

Just pop this baby in the oven while you're blow-drying your mess and then take it on the road. Delicious organic potatoes, tofu, black beans, vegetables, and salsa stuffed into an organic flour tortilla (amys.com).

Stir-Fries

Stir-fries are like a hodgepodge of happiness. You get a little bit of everything, all those different flavors competing for recognition in your mouth. But you know what I don't want competing in my mouth? Preservatives, GMOs, artificial dyes, added MSG, and trans fats. Sewer water sounds more appetizing than that.

Instead of diddle-daddling in the frozen-food aisle freezing your nipples off, know what you're looking for before you enter the tundra. These frozen entrees are made with healthy ingredients, such as organic vegetables, spices, herbs, nuts, and seeds that have been nurtured by Mother Earth, without the added junk.

*Amy's Thai Stir-fry

Organic cabbage, carrots, zucchini, jalapenos, mixed bell peppers, jasmine rice, and tofu coated in a coconut-milk sauce with pure herbs and spices (amys.com).

Kashi Black Bean Mango Frozen Entree

Black beans, red onions, green peppers, and carrots all roasted, grilled, and seasoned to bring out the rich flavors. Served on a bed of Kashi's signature 7 Whole Grain Pilaf with a spicy mango sauce (kashi.com).

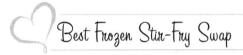
Best Frozen Stir-Fry Swap

Moo Moo's Cuisine Roasted Cashew Stir-Fry

A mixture of whole-grain noodles with cabbage, scallions, red bell peppers, pineapple, and roasted cashews and sesame seeds in a special brown sauce (moomooscuisine.com).

*Amy's Brown Rice and Vegetable Bowl

Organic brown rice, onions, mushrooms, carrots, spinach, broccoli, and marinated tofu in a sesame tahini sauce (amys.com).

*Amy's Light in Sodium Brown Rice and Vegetables Bowl

The twin sister of the Brown Rice and Vegetables Bowl, but with half the sodium (amys.com).

Swap that ‿‿‿‿‿

Rice Gourmet Grilled Chicken Teriyaki Bowl

‿‿‿‿‿ for this

*Amy's Teriyaki Bowl

Assorted veggies, herbs, spices, and marinated tofu on organic brown rice in a sweet teriyaki sauce (amys.com).

*Amy's Asian Noodle Stir-Fry

Organic noodles, tofu, broccoli, carrots, bell peppers, and mushrooms tossed in a tangy ginger garlic sauce (amys.com).

Best Surprisingly Addictive Swap

Morningstar Farms Sesame Chik'n

Breaded veggie "chicken," sugar snap peas, carrots, and red peppers over Asian noodles in a sesame sauce. It's surprisingly low in calories but doesn't earn five stars in the sodium category, so eat responsibly (morningstarfarms.com).

Morningstar Farms Sweet and Sour Chik'n

Breaded veggie "chicken," pineapple, carrots, and red and green bell peppers on whole-grain rice. Panda Express would be jealous of this sweet-and-sour dish, and it didn't have to while away the hours on a buffet line all day (morningstarfarms.com).

Entrees

*Sukhi's Vegan Chili Chicken

Vegan soy "chicken" dunked in an Indian chili sauce with bell peppers, onion, tomatoes, ginger, garlic, and spices. Served with naan bread (sukhis.com).

*Amy's Baked Ziti Bowl

Baked rice pasta topped with organic peas, soy cheeses, and an Italian herb pasta sauce that has Amy's written all over it (amys.com).

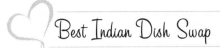

Best Indian Dish Swap

*Amy's Indian Mattar Tofu

A vegan twist on the traditional Indian dish, with tofu and organic peas in a flavorful sauce. Served with basmati rice and Amy's version of lentil dal (amys.com).

*Amy's Black Bean Vegetable Enchilada

Organic black beans, tofu, and a medley of veggies rolled up in two organic corn tortillas covered in enchilada sauce (amys.com).

*Amy's Mexican Tamale Pie

A polenta pie filled with organic corn, zucchini, pinto beans, and onions simmered in a Mexican sauce (amys.com).

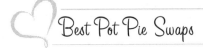

Best Pot Pie Swaps

*Amy's Shepherd's Pie and Amy's Vegetable Pot Pie

I really couldn't choose between these two—they are both so equally delicious. A popular Irish dish minus the meat, the Shepherd's Pie is a warm blanket of mashed potatoes and organic vegetables in a savory broth (also available in Light in Sodium). The Vegetable Pot Pie is made with organic carrots, peas, potatoes, and tofu in a thick, creamy sauce (amys.com).

*Amy's Dairy Free Rice Macaroni and Cheeze

Organic rice macaroni smothered in Amy's nondairy cheeze (amys.com).

Kashi Mayan Harvest Bake

A totally unique dish with plantains, sweet potatoes, black beans, and kale over Kashi 7 Whole Grain Polenta in a hot ancho sauce. Then I get done in by the pinch of pumpkin seeds over the top (kashi.com).

Best Steak Swap

Vegetarian Plus Vegan Black Pepper Steaks

You can have your tri-tip and eat it too. The texture and flavor of these low-in-sodium pepper steaks scream gourmet. They have a spicy, peppery kick with just the right amount of sweetness (vegeusa.com).

Best "Takeout" Swap

Trader Joe's Vegan Pad Thai with Tofu

Quickie Thai rice noodles in a fun Chinese takeout box—perfect for the dorm room or a meal on the go. Just open up the box, tear open the sauce packets, mix it all up, and microwave it right in the carton.

It's a slightly different twist on traditional pad thai, but the flavors are flippin' awesome. It never gets old (traderjoes.com).

*Moo Moo's Cuisine Poblano Chick(Pea) Patties

No guessing what's inside. Just chick peas, chili onions, brown rice, and roasted bell and poblano peppers mashed into patties. Served with corn salsa (moomooscuisine.com).

*Moo Moo's Cuisine Black Bean Cakes and Mango Slaw

Mashed patties made of black beans, brown rice, roasted bell peppers, caramelized onions, and cranberries kettle-cooked with Caribbean flair (moomooscuisine.com).

*Moo Moo's Cuisine Sweet 'N Spicy Curry Tofu

Break the everyday monotony with marinated organic tofu blended in a zesty curry sauce with raisins, cabbage, pineapple, and sesame seeds (moomooscuisine.com).

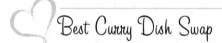

Best Curry Dish Swap

Helen's Kitchen Thai Yellow Curry with Tofu Steaks and Vegetables over Basmati Rice

I think this speaks for itself, but this medley of vegetables and certi-fied organic ingredients puts me in travel mode every time. It's full of chunks of tofu and broccoli over rice in an exotic curry sauce. I fill my freezer with these just in case I need something quick and gourmet (thehelenskitchen.com).

Helen's Kitchen Indian Curry with Tofu Steaks over Rice

Authentic Indian flavor, with certified organic herbs and spices (the helenskitchen.com).

Helen's Kitchen Thai Red Curry

Organic green peas, butternut squash, and red bell peppers over basmati rice (thehelenskitchen.com).

Trader Joe's Misto Alla Griglia

Marinated grilled eggplant and zucchini you can add to stir-fries, sandwiches, wraps, and casseroles (traderjoes.com).

Best Pasta Dish Swap

Trader Joe's Penne Arriabbiata

Just add a few tablespoons of oil to the skillet, empty in this frozen bag of pasta, and you've got an Italian pasta dinner in minutes. Hearty tomato and onion make this an authentic Italian meal that tastes like you made it from scratch (traderjoes.com).

Pizza

A pizza without cheese is like a hotel room without a mirror above the bed—no fun at all. But it turns out that's a big, fat misconception (talking about the pizza). There are dozens of vegan food brands that know just how to make the right slice with or without the (vegan) cheese. Some go as far to pleasure us with plant-based toppings such as pepperoni and sausage. Mmmm . . .

Swap that ～～～

～～～ for this

Tofurky Cheese Pizza

If there is one marriage that can survive the bumps in the road, it's Tofurky and Daiya Cheese. The guys who gave birth to the fake turkey took a thin, flaky, whole-wheat crust and topped it with a garlic tomato pizza sauce and gooey, melted soy cheese for the best damn vegan cheese pizza I've ever had. Suck it, Dominos (tofurky.com).

Best Transition Pizza
Best Swap for a Meat Lover's Pizza Party

Tofurky "Meat" Pizzas

Choose between Tofurky's Pepperoni Pizza and its Italian Sausage Pizza, which is dressed up with soy sausage, sun-dried tomatoes, basil, and Daiya cheese (tofurky.com).

⫘➡ *Tofurky isn't selfish when it comes to the toppings. If you get a variety other than the traditional cheese, you'll find it piled high!*

American Flatbread Vegan Harvest Pizza

Flatbread dough topped with organic tomato sauce, herbs, and of course Daiya's mozzarella cheese (americanflatbread.com).

Amy's Roasted Vegetable Pizza

No cheese, only marinated artichoke hearts, organic shiitake mushrooms, roasted red peppers, and sweet onions on a wheat-flour crust (amys.com).

*Amy's Rice Crust Spinach Pizza

A thin rice crust covered with organic spinach, soy-based mozzarella and ricotta cheeses, and Amy's signature pizza sauce (amys.com).

*Amy's Single Serve Rice Crust Roasted Vegetable Pizza

A replica of the Roasted Vegetable Pizza, but gluten-free on a rice crust. Made specially for one (amys.com).

Best Gluten-Free Swap

*Amy's Single Serve Non-Dairy Rice Crust Cheese Pizza

A simple, gluten-free "cheese" pizza for one with a crispy crust that is similar to cornmeal, but without the corn taste. It's pretty basic, but my hubby knows how to jazz it up with some herbs and premium olive oil before baking. Keep in mind, the cheese will only melt if you put it in the toaster oven or broiler for the last minute of baking, but it's worth the extra step (amys.com).

Tofutti Pan Crust Pizza Pizzaz

Perfect for one, Tofutti's pizza is drizzled with a tomato sauce and vegan mozzarella on a pan-style crust (tofutti.com).

Rossini's Gourmet Vegan Pizzas

Daiya Italian and cheddar cheeses melted on a medium-thick crust. Choose from Cheese, Pepperoni (with Yves vegan pepperoni), and Italian Sausage (with Upton's sausage-flavored seitan crumbles; store .veganessentials.com).

Best "Veggie Only" Swap

Trader Joe's Vegan Roasted Vegetable Pizza

An organic, crisp wheat-flour crust dressed with caramelized onions, artichokes, and shiitake mushrooms. An exquisite pizza at an even more exquisite price (traderjoes.com).

Swap that ༼

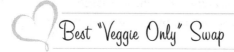

Stouffer's French Bread Pizza

for this

*Ian's Vegan French Bread Pizza

A gluten-free French bread pizza with a hearty Italian sauce and soy mozzarella cheese. In my book, there's nothing better than a French bread pizza for an in-between meal. It's best to pop this one in the toaster oven so the cheese melts quickly (iansnaturalfoods.com).

Appetizers

Best Indian Appetizer Swap

Sukhi's Vegan Samosas and Chutney

Crispy on the outside and tender on the inside, these samosas are stuffed with plump chunks of spiced potatoes and peas in a cilantro chutney (sukhis.com).

Trader Joe's Meatless Meatballs

No MSG or artificial colors or flavors—just drizzle some tomato sauce on top and you're golden (traderjoes.com).

Swap that

Frozen meatballs

for this

Nate's Meatless Meatballs

These are easy to prepare and so versatile. Heat them up for some spaghetti or stick some toothpicks in 'em for an appetizer. They come in three delicious flavors: Classic, Zesty Italian, and Savory Mushroom (foodservicedirect.com).

KIM'S PICK: The Classic variety has a mild, peppery flavor, but it takes on the taste of whatever it's cooked with.

Best Dumpling Swap

Trader Joe's Thai Vegetable Gyoza

Instead of in the traditional thick dough made with egg, these steamed dumplings are wrapped in wonton wrappers; the filling features cabbage, carrots, chives, radishes, garlic, and ginger. They're the perfect appetizer (traderjoes.com).

➡ *Entertaining on a budget? Just heat these up and serve in a dish for a light appetizer that costs next to nothing.*

Health Is Wealth Vegan Vegetable Potstickers

All natural ingredients packed tightly in wheat dumplings. Whether you're into the "Pork-Free" or the "Chicken-Free" style, expect true-to-form taste and texture (healthiswealthfoods.com).

Health Is Wealth Vegan Veggie Munchies

Assorted veggies wrapped in bite-size mini shells made of whole wheat and expeller-pressed nonhydrogenated oils. No MSG, preservatives, or trans fats (healthiswealthfoods.com).

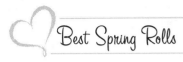 Best Spring Rolls

Health Is Wealth Vegan Vegetable Spring Rolls

These taste just like the traditional spring rolls you would order at your neighborhood Chinese restaurant, but there's no meat in these crispy, juicy delights. Each roll is stuffed with tofu and veggies, with no MSG or any artificial additives, colors, flavors, and preservatives (healthiswealthfoods.com).

> *Try them with Trader Joe's San Soyaki Sauce, a bold teriyaki dipping sauce and marinade that adds instant flavor.*

Health Is Wealth Vegan Thai Spring Rolls

Wheat pastries filled with cabbage, carrots, onions, rice noodles, mushrooms, and marinated tofu in a Thai peanut sauce (healthiswealth foods.com).

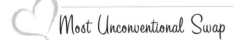 Most Unconventional Swap

VegeCyber Vegan Crab Meat Balls

Eat these à la carte with a sweet-and-sour dipping sauce or add to BBQ dishes, stir-fries, soups, and noodles (vegecyber.com).

fat
fact

Want a good reason to go vegan? Just one vegan spares 198 animals from slaughter at a factory farm.

Dessert and Baking Swaps

Cookies

Oreos, Chips Ahoy, Fig Newtons, Pepperidge Farm Milanos—you know these guys better than you know your own mother. Here are a few better, healthier alternatives with no cholesterol, artificial flavors, colors, preservatives, or scary ingredients that come from animals. They are all living proof that your sweet tooth doesn't have to suffer because you actually care about your health.

Liz Lovely Vegan Cookies

Ride 'em, cowgirl! Made with vegan, organic ingredients, these dee-lish cookies keep me from stalking Girl Scouts. They come in dozens of flavors including Cowboy Cookies (with walnuts, oats, and chocolate chips), Cowgirl Cookies (chocolate chip, with dark chocolate drizzled on top), Ginger Snapdragons, Peanut Butter Classics, Chocolate Moose Dragons, Snicker Dudes, and many more (lizlovely.com).

Laura's Wholesome Junk Food Cookies

Like your obsession with reality TV, these are just plain dangerous. But they are completely natural and made in the U.S.A., so screw it. Available in Oatmeal Chocolate Chip, Oatmeal Raisin, Xtreme Chocolate Fudge, Better Brownie, Anna-Banana Split, Cole's Cashew Chocolate Chip, Lemon-Vanilla, Mint Double Fudge, Grandma's Gingerbread, and Cranberry Breakfast (lauraswholesomejunkfood.com).

*Nana's Cookie Company Cookies

Individually wrapped cookies, cookie bites, and cookie bars sweetened with fruit juices. Available in Double Chocolate, Oatmeal Raisin, Peanut Butter, Coconut Chip, Chocolate Chip. Gluten Free available in Lemon, Ginger, Chocolate, and Chocolate Crunch. No Wheat available in Chocolate Chip and Oatmeal Raisin (nanascookiecompany.com).

Michelle's Naturally Cookies

Born and raised in South America, Michelle, a California-based baker, grew up experimenting with spices and flavorings. Now she sells her fruit juice–sweetened cookies through natural-food stores. They are truly addictive. Available in Chocolate Chip, Rainforest Oatmeal Raisin, Peanut Butter Apricot, Almond Dot Poppyseed, Oatmeal Cranberry Passion, Chocolate Chip Oatmeal, Chocolate Chip Pe-

An asterisk (*) means the product is gluten-free.

can, Chocolate Chip Peanut Butter, and Gluten Free Chocolate Chip (michellesnaturally.com).

Swap that ∽∽∿⤵

⤸∽∽∽ *for this*

Late July Organic Sandwich Cookies

Made with whole grains and no artificial crap. Available in Vanilla Bean with Green Tea, and Dark Chocolate (latejuly.com).

Make Your Own (or Eat It Raw)

Bake your own with EatPastry's Cookie Dough in six delectable flavors. EatPastry doesn't mess around with animal ingredients or artificial sugars. Expect organic and fair-trade evaporated cane juice and other organic ingredients that haven't been put through the ringer with fillers, GMOs, or preservatives. If you're not the baking type, it's also tasty (and safe) to eat raw, straight out of the carton (the perfect cure for PMS).

Available in the refrigerator section in Chocolate Chunk (also in gluten-free), Peanut Butter, Ginger, Oatmeal Raisin, and Chocoholic Chunk. Visit eatpastry.com for more cookies du jour.

Newman-O's Crème Filled Cookies

Cookies made with organic unbleached flour and no partially hydrogenated oils—only an organic icing center. Try the Original flavor if you're looking for the best Oreo swap. Available in Original, Chocolate, Peanut Butter, Ginger 'N Crème, Dairy Free Crème, and Hint-O-Mint (newmansownorganics.com).

Swap that ᗛᗝᗝᗝᗛ

Nabisco Chips Ahoy

ᗛᗝᗝᗝᗝ *for this*

Back to Nature Chocolate Chunk Cookies

These are actually bigger, better, and chunkier than Chips Ahoy, with more of a homemade quality and no hydrogenated oils or fake ingredients or colors. We're talking serious chunks of chocolate! Dip them in almond milk for an intense experience (backtonaturefoods.com).

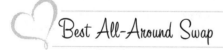 *Best All-Around Swap*

Uncle Eddies Vegan Cookies

Cross my heart and hope to die, you will never know these babies are vegan. They are made with nothing but simple ingredients that you would find in your own pantry (not in a laboratory). They are my husband's favorite cookies (bastard's not vegan), and I can even feel comfortable feeding half a box to my son (little dude has me wrapped around his damn finger). Did I mention that the company supports sustainable agriculture, bakes with organic and fair-trade ingredients, and packages its products in environmentally friendly packaging? I'll shut up now. Available in Chocolate Chip with Walnuts, Oatmeal Chocolate Chip, Trail Mix, Oatmeal Raisin, Cocoa Spice and Everything Nice, Peanut Butter Chocolate Chip, and Molasses (uncleeddiesvegancookies.com).

*Dr. Lucy's Cookies

Got allergies? Dr. Lucy's ensures that no peanuts, tree nuts, milk, or eggs even come close to its bite-size treats. And for all you bitches who can't live without your morning Starbucks run, you can find Dr. Lucy's right in the coffee shop's baked goods section. Available in Chocolate Chip, Cinnamon Thin (think Snickerdoodle), Sugar, and Oatmeal (drlucys.com).

Ice Cream

I scream, you scream, we all scream for what?! Butter, cream, milk, egg yolks, partially hydrogenated oils, and corn syrup? No, thank you, Ben & Jerry's. Here's the scoop: vegan ice cream has come a *l-o-n-g* way. You name the flavor, and there's a better knockoff.

Best Coconut Milk Ice Cream Swap

*Luna and Larry's Organic Coconut Bliss

If the ice cream truck in my neighborhood carried these pints, I would have begged my parents for more chores. Each original flavor is whipped up with coconut milk, which gives it a sweet, delicate flavor and texture without the soy or gluten. If you're afraid you'll finish the whole carton watching Twilight on HBO, they also carry ice cream bars. Flavors available in Naked Almond Fudge, Naked Coconut, Pineapple Coconut, Mocha Maca Crunch, Ginger Cookie Caramel, Chocolate Walnut Brownie, Lunaberry Swirl, Chocolate Peanut Butter, Dark Chocolate, Vanilla Island, Mint Galactica, Cappuccino, Cherry Amaretto, and Chocolate Hazelnut Fudge (coconutbliss.com).

KIM'S PICK: No matter how much I try to change it up, I always grab the Cherry Amaretto, which boasts a plentiful mix of cherries and almond flavor.

Swap that ⟳⟳⟳⟳

Sorbet

⟳⟳⟳⟳ for this

Sharon's Sorbet

Holy shit, Batman, this stuff is good. It has the perfect texture and only a few simple raw ingredients. Lucky for us, it's cheap and easy to find at major grocery retailers. Available in Strawberry, Coconut, Mango, Lemon, Dutch Chocolate, Mixed Berry, Passion Fruit, Blueberry, and Raspberry (sharons-sorbet.com).

KIM'S PICK: Lemon Sorbet.

Double Rainbow Gourmet Soy Cream and Sorbet

Irresistible soy cream and sorbet pints full of flavor. The founders chose their name after seeing a double rainbow the day after signing the lease on their first ice cream parlor. It's like eating a scoop of good karma. Soy cream available in Blueberry, Cinnamon Caramel, Mint Chocolate Chip, Vanilla Bean, and Very Cherry Chip. Gluten-free, fruit-based sorbet available in Chocolate, Coconut, Lemon, Mango Tangerine, and Raspberry (doublerainbow.com).

Turtle Mountain So Delicious Ice Cream

Take your pick from coconut- or soy-based, dairy-free ice cream and ice cream novelties (bars and sandwiches) in tons of flavors. Quart flavors available in Chocolate Peanut Butter, Chocolate Velvet, Cookies 'N Cream, Creamy Vanilla, Mint Marble Fudge, Mocha Fudge, Neapolitan, and Strawberry. Fruit-sweetened pints available in Almond Pecan, Awesome Chocolate, Black Leopard, Carob Peppermint, Chocolate Almond, Chocolate Peanut Butter, Espresso, Green Tea, Mango Raspberry, Pistachio Almond, Raspberry, Tiger Chai, Vanilla, and Vanilla Fudge (turtlemountain.com).

Novelty Ice Cream Bars available in Creamy Fudge Bar (organic), Chocolate Sandwich (organic), Mint Sandwich (organic), Neapolitan Sandwich (organic), Vanilla Sandwich (organic), Creamy Vanilla Bar

Kids' Classics:
Dairy-Free Alternatives to the Treats We'll Never Get Too Old For

Swap that: **Ice cream sandwich**
for this: **Turtle Mountain So Delicious Organic Vanilla Sandwich**
Ice cream packed between two delicious chocolate cakes. Also comes in Chocolate, Mint, and Neapolitan (turtlemountain.com).

Swap that: **Fudgesicle**
for this: **Turtle Mountain So Delicious Organic Creamy Fudge Bar**
Rich, creamy chocolate on a stick—just like the fudge bars we ate as kids (turtlemountain.com).

Best Chocolate Chip Sandwich Swap
Turtle Mountain So Delicious Chocolate Chip Sandwich
If you're looking for something beyond the norm, this is like a chocolate chip cookie mash-up. Fun for the whole fam (turtlemountain.com).

(organic), Creamy Raspberry Bar, Creamy Orange Bar, Chocolate Minis Sandwich, Mint Minis Sandwich, Neapolitan Minis Sandwich, Orange Passion Fruit Minis Fruit Bar, Pomegranate Minis Sandwich, Vanilla and Almonds Bar (organic), Raspberry Minis Fruit Bar, Strawberry Minis Fruit Bar, and Vanilla Minis Sandwich.

Fruit Sweetened Pints available in Almond Pecan, Awesome Chocolate, Black Leopard, Carob Peppermint, Chocolate Almond, Chocolate Peanut Butter, Espresso, Green Tea, Mango Raspberry, Pistachio Almond, Raspberry, Tiger Chai, Vanilla, and Vanilla Fudge.

Ice Cream Novelties with Coconut Milk available in Banana Split Minis Sandwich, Chocolate Almond Minis Sandwich, Coconut Minis Sandwich, and Vanilla Minis Bar.

Novelties available in Chocolate Chip Sandwich, Creamy Fudge Bar, and Mint Chocolate Chip Sandwich.

Kidz Assorted Fruit Pops available in Fudge Bar, Sweet Nothings Fudge Bar, and Sweet Nothings Mango Raspberry Bar.

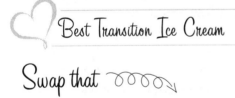

Best Transition Ice Cream

Swap that ༽

Baskin-Robbins Ice Cream

for this

Turtle Mountain Purely Decadent Ice Cream

The crème de la crème of vegan ice creams, Purely Decadent is a line of soy-based, dairy-free ice creams that have a creamier, richer texture and flavor. They're higher in fat, but still have less fat than the dairy-filled ice creams. There are tons of great flavors—like, for example, Blueberry Cheesecake, Cherry Nirvana, Dulce de Leche, Key Lime Pie, Pomegranate Chip, Praline Pecan, Snickerdoodle, and Turtle Trails—but my ultimate favorite is the Mocha Almond Fudge. Soy-free coconut-milk varieties include Chocolate, Chocolate Peanut Butter Swirl, Coconut, Mocha Almond Fudge, Passionate Mango, Vanilla Bean, and more.

Baking Mixes

Betty and Duncan may know how to make a damn good cake, but God forbid they throw anything slightly healthy in the mix. Just take a gander at some of the ingredients in Betty Crocker and Duncan Hines cake mixes: bleached flour, sugar, corn syrup, partially hydrogenated soybean oil, modified corn starch (hello, GMOs?!), animal fatty acids, sodium stearoyl lactylate, propylene glycol (um, why?), and artificial flavors. Sorry, but I'm not down with these ingredients (nor do I feel like grabbing a dictionary for help).

Since I'm a baker at heart, I like to make everything from scratch, but it's always great to have a few mixes on hand, so I can whip up a treat in a jiffy—especially for those few days a month when I turn into Satan's sister and would give a kidney for some dessert.

These mixes are made with simple, healthier alternatives that I could find in my own pantry. Now tell me, Betty . . . is it really that tough?

*Pure Pantry Mixes

Gluten-free baking mixes that use only natural, certified organic ingredients that come from whole grains. Not just for cakes, but pancakes and cookies too. Available in Organic Old Fashioned Pancake and Baking Mix, Organic Buckwheat Flax Pancake and Baking Mix, Organic All-Purpose Baking Mix, Old Fashioned Chocolate Chip Cookie Mix, and Wholegrain Dark Chocolate Cake Mix (thepure pantry.com).

Best Transition Baking Mixes

Swap that

Duncan Hines Baking Mixes

for this

*Cherrybrook Kitchen Baking Mixes

Cherrybrook knows what a vegan wants her vegan cakes and cookies to taste like. Its all-natural baking mixes are free of peanuts, dairy, eggs, and nuts, and some are wheat- or gluten-free. They are quick and easy to make, with a moist fluffiness that is tough to come by in cruelty-free baking. Even the gluten-free version knocked my socks off. My favorites are the Fudge Brownie, Chocolate Cake, and Original Pancake Mix. Mixes also available in Sugar Cookie and Chocolate Chip Cookie (cherrybrookkitchen.com).

> *Refrigerator note: If any mix calls for an egg, don't lose your shit. Just swap it out for egg replacer.*

*Wholesome Chow Mixes

All you need is a milk alternative and some vinegar to turn one of these mixes into a velvety cake. The lavender flavor is subtle but amazing, and the Chai Spice Cake is exotic with bursts of cardamom, nutmeg, and ginger. Mixes available in Decadent Chocolate Cake, Vivacious Vanilla Cake, Luscious Lavender Cake, Lively Chai Spice Cake, Gluten Free Chocolate Cake, Gluten Free Chocolate Lavender Cake, Gluten Free Chocolate Spice Cake, and Vegan Homestyle Cornbread (wholesomechow.com).

Dr. Oetker Organics Baking Mixes

A doctor with all the goods, Dr. Oetker ensures every ingredient used is grown pesticide- and chemical-free. Mixes available in Pancake and Waffle, Chocolate Chip Cookie, Oatmeal Cookie, Chocolate Brownie, Marble Cake, Vanilla Cake, and Chocolate Cake (oetker.us).

*Simply Organic Baking Mixes

Certified organic and gluten-free baking mixes made with wholesome ingredients. Try the Carrot Cake and Banana Bread mixes (simply organicfoods.com).

Sugar

Artificial sugar is like liquid crack. The processed shit in Equal, Sweet'N Low, and Splenda raises our insulin levels, wears down our immune systems, makes us susceptible to diseases, and turns us into lard asses.

Whether we like it or not, Americans consume about two to three pounds of sugar a week! Food manufacturers add it to everyday foods like gravy, pasta, and salad dressings to boost the flavor. With that said, not only do you want to look for healthier sweeteners in prepackaged foods—such as evaporated cane sugar, stevia, agave nectar, and Sucanat—but you want to make sure this is the stuff you're using in your own kitchen. Quit listening to your grandma . . . she's senile anyway.

Hollah! Vegan Staple

Evaporated Cane Sugar

Best Transition Sugar   Best Everyday Sugar Swap

Florida Crystals Organic Cane Sugar

Certified organic, natural cane sugar that tastes pretty damn close to white table sugar. I use it as an everyday cane sugar sweetener for tea, cereals, desserts, and whatever else calls for a boost. Also comes in Demerara Sugar, with a hint of molasses in each crystal (florida crystals.com).

O Organics Organic Evaporated Cane Juice Sugar

Crystallized within twenty-four hours of harvesting, O Organics evaporated cane sugar is certified organic by the USDA (safeway.com).

Bob's Red Mill Evaporated Cane Juice Sugar

All-natural cane sugar with no additives (bobsredmill.com).

*Navitas Naturals Sweet Tooth Organic Evaporated Palm Sugar

A certified organic, gourmet-style sugar made from plant-based ingredients that is safe for diabetics; it's low on the glycemic index and low in calories (navitasnaturals.com).

India Tree Gourmet Spices and Specialties Demerara Sugar

A raw, golden cane-style sugar with underlying spice and buttery tones (indiatree.com).

*Big Tree Farms SweetTree Organic Coconut Palm Sugar, Blonde

Gaining some steam in the health world as the new alternative sugar of choice, coconut-palm sugar has a soft caramel flavor reminiscent of light brown sugar. This unrefined sugar is high in nutrients, boasts a low number on the glycemic index, and is brought to you by local artisans fighting to sustain the culturally rich islands of Indonesia (bigtreebali.com).

Shady Maple Farms Certified Organic Pure Maple Sugar

One hundred percent natural and organic maple sugar with no additives (amazon.com).

Billington's Natural Demerara Unrefined Cane Sugar

Billington's is known for its high-quality golden baking sugars. If you're a coffee drinker, then this is your poison (billingtons.co.uk).

Essential Living Foods Palm Flower Nectar Coconut Sugar

Widely available at stores nationwide, this organic cane sugar alternative is grown and harvested by small farms with 100 percent of the proceeds going back to the local community. For all my tree huggers, it even comes in biodegradable packaging. Score (essentialliving foods.com).

Brown Sugar and Syrups

Navitas Naturals Sweet Tooth Organic Yacon Syrup

Derived from the sweet roots of South American plant that looks like a jicama, but tastes like molasses, yacon syrup has half the calories of cane sugar. A safe alternative for diabetics (navitasnaturals.com).

TerrAmazon Organic Raw Premium Yacon Syrup

Easy on your digestive system, TerrAmazon's yacon sugar comes in a syrup or semidried slices for snacking (terramazon.com).

Lundberg Organic Sweet Dreams Brown Rice Syrup

For those watching their sugar intake, Lundberg's brown rice syrup is half as sweet as sugar (lundberg.com).

Eden Organic Traditional Barley Malt Syrup

Great for baking spice cakes, gingerbread, homemade BBQ sauces, and baked beans, this thick, dark brown syrup is nothin' but barley and water. Clean as a whistle (edenfoods.com).

Plantation Blackstrap Unsulphured Molasses

Loaded with potassium, blackstrap molasses is the thickest, darkest, and most mineral-dense form of molasses. Some claim this reverses their gray hair (alliedoldenglish.com).

365 Everyday Value Organic Raw Agave Nectar

With a scent and taste similar to honey, Whole Foods' signature agave nectar is great for sweetening beverages (wholefoodsmarket.com).

Nature's Agave Raw 100% Organic Premium Blue Agave

Choose from three organic varieties harvested from the Weber Blue Agave plant. No chemicals or additives are added to the mix (natures agave.com).

Maple Syrups

There is a reason pancake maple syrup tastes and looks cheap. It's just a plastic squeeze bottle of high-fructose corn syrup, preservatives, artificial flavors, and almost no genuine maple content. And there is absolutely no stinkin' way to tell if it's vegan, because who knows how it's processed? Maple syrup, on the other hand, is the real dealio. Make sure to buy 100 percent pure maple syrup, because other grades go through a defoaming process that adds a smidgen of fat to the syrup. All of the products below are healthier alternatives for pancakes and waffles, with a deep, rich flavor and texture.

Trader Joe's Maple Syrup

Available in 100% Pure Vermont Grade A Maple Syrup, Organic Maple Syrup, and Organic Maple Agave Blend (traderjoes.com).

NOW Organic 100% Pure Maple Syrup

(nowfoods.com)

Pure & Natural Vermont Grade B Maple Syrup

(piecesofvermont.com)

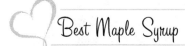

Best Maple Syrup

Shady Maple Farms Certified Organic Pure Maple Syrup

Rich maple flavor, and a consistency that isn't too thick or thin. Great for baking too (amazon.com).

Fresh & Easy Organic 100% Pure Vermont Maple Syrup

(freshandeasy.com)

365 Organic 100% Pure Grade B Maple Syrup

(wholefoodsmarket.com)

— THE SKINNY —

Wholesome Sweeteners

Wholesome Sweeteners is your one-stop shoppe for everything sugar. Whether you're a baker, a sugar aficionado, or just want to wake up your iced tea, Whole Sweeteners offers more than twenty different organic sugar varieties that are certified fair trade. Choose from the likes of Organic Raw Blue Agave, Organic Sucanat, Organic Light Brown Sugar, and Organic Powdered Sugar. It also offers Organic Zero Packets, a sugar substitute that is not quite as sweet as sugar, with no calories and a reading of 0 on the glycemic index. Say good-bye to spikes to your blood sugar. Available at Costco, Trader Joe's, and Whole Foods and online at wholesomesweeteners.com.

Stevia

*Navitas Naturals Sweet Tooth Organic Raw Stevia Powder

The third product in the Sweet Tooth line, Navitas Naturals' stevia powder is made from the whole leaves of the stevia plant, undergoing no processing. You only need a pinch—stevia is three hundred times sweeter than sugar, yet it won't spike insulin levels (navitas naturals.com).

SweetLeaf Stevia Packets

All-natural stevia free from chemicals or nasty additives. Carry these packets in your purse for beverages on the go (sweetleaf.com).

*NOW BetterStevia Packets

Now uses the whole-leaf extract to retain stevia's pure, clean sweetness. Certified organic by the USDA, with no artificial ingredients (nowfoods.com).

Flours and Meals

Flour looks all innocent and wholesome, but the stuff you find in your everyday grocery hell is bleached and whitened with chemicals such as potassium bromate and benzoyl peroxide. Yeah, it's no good. Stick to unrefined, unbleached brands in different varieties such as all-purpose, whole wheat, whole grain, or buckwheat (gluten-free). As with everything, try to buy organic to make sure the grain has been grown without the use of synthetic pesticides, fertilizers, or GMOs.

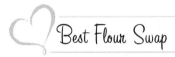
Best Flour Swap

*King Arthur Flours

King Arthur is the queen of options, with premium, unbleached flours milled fresh from wheat berries. They're available just about anywhere and make great pancakes, biscuits, and desserts. Available in All-Purpose, Bread, White Whole Wheat, Whole Wheat, Cake, Spelt, Barley, Gluten-Free, and more. King Arthur also offers stone-ground Organic Yellow Cornmeal, ideal for making muffins, bread, and cornbread (kingarthurflour.com).

*Arrowhead Mills Flours

This all-natural line of whole-grain specialty flours keeps all cooking preferences and allergies in mind with twenty different varieties (arrowheadmills.com).

*Bob's Red Mill Flours

Bob's unbleached, whole-grain flours in white or wheat, meals, and pastry flours are fitting for everyday cooking (bobsredmill.com).

*Let's Do . . . Organic Coconut Flour

High in fiber, low in fat, and gluten-free, this flour is made from organic coconut. A superb alternative to wheat. Also try the Organic Cornstarch or Organic Tapioca Starch (edwardandsons.com).

Icing

Spread it on thick, honey. These icings contain simpler ingredients, such as cocoa powder, soybean oil, and natural vanilla flavor, so you can feel comfortable licking the spoon. Traditional ingredients in frosting aren't quite as lickable. We're talking modified corn starch, artificial flavor, gelatin, egg whites, and sodium lauryl sulfate (yes, SLS is indeed hiding in a can of one of Betty Crocker's frosting mixes). Yuck! Make the swap for something that's cake-worthy.

Swap that ༠༠༠༠

Betty Crocker Frosting

༠༠༠༠ for this

*Cherrybrook Kitchen Frosting

Whether you like making it yourself or just want something that requires as little effort as possible 'cause you're a lazy ass, Cherrybrook carries a ready-made spread and frosting mixes. These are packaged mixes, so all you need to do is add a milk alternative and some Earth Balance and whip away for a creamy, fluffy frosting that's sex on a stick. They have the best flavor, and the Earth Balance really helps up the creamy quotient. All varieties are nut- and gluten-free. Available in Vanilla Frosting Ready to Spread, and as a mix in Chocolate Frosting and Vanilla Frosting (cherrybrookkitchen.com).

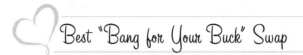
Best "Bang for Your Buck" Swap

Trader Joe's Baker Josef's Frosting Mix

You just have to add hot water and a tablespoon of Earth Balance and mix with an electric mixer. A sweet, healthy alternative with a smooth flavor. Available in White and Chocolate (traderjoes.com).

Dr. Oetker Organics Icing Mixes

These all-natural mixes turn out just as rich and creamy as dairy mixes, and they've gone through no chemical processing. Mixes available in Vanilla Icing and Chocolate Icing (oetker.us).

Pudding and Gels

There's just something about those little plastic cups of joy that make me wish I was a kid again. I remember staring at the clock in grade school, just waiting for the lunch bell to ring, so I could dig into that creamy or jiggly filling. Well, some things never change. The only difference is that now I'm usually stealing them from my kid's lunchbox (don't worry, I replace with an apple). Nowadays, these are the brands I turn to rather than filling up on artificial ingredients and animal gelatin.

Pudding

Swap that ∿∿∿

Jell-O Pudding

∿∿∿ *for this*

*Zen Organic Soy Pudding

Made from organic soybeans grown in the United States, these gluten-free pudding packs are wonderfully creamy and smooth. Available in Vanilla, Chocolate, Banana, and Chocolate/Vanilla Swirl (zensoy.com).

Gels

Swap that ∿∿∿

Jell-O

∿∿∿ *for this*

Cool Cups Natural Snacks

Fat- and gluten-free, these gel cups are chock-full of vitamin C. And they are pretty darn close to real Jell-O, despite not having any gelatin to give them that wiggly but firm consistency. My son won't let me leave the grocery store without the Orange and Black Cherry. Gels available in Natural Orange, Natural Black Cherry, and Natural Peach (cool-cups.com).

*Trader Joe's Natural Gel Cups

These cups are fluffier and almost dissolve in your mouth with non-gelatin jiggle. Fat- and gluten-free. Available in Peach Mango and Black Cherry (traderjoes.com).

Pudding Mix

Mmmm . . . cream-filled pies. So yummy and filling. These mixes are great for making lush pie and pastry fillings or for whipping up to eat alone with a dollop of soy whipped cream. Nobody's judging.

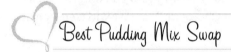

Best Pudding Mix Swap

Dr. Oetker Organics Pudding Mixes

Just add your favorite milk alternative, cook, and melt. They don't quite thicken enough for my liking, but they are great to add to other ingredients to make desserts. I add them to my cake batters to get a moist consistency, and it works like a gem. Organic mixes available in Chocolate, Banana, Coconut, Vanilla, and Butterscotch (oetker.us).

Mori-Nu Mates Low-Fat Pudding Mixes

Easy to whip up. Just blend with some silken lite tofu and you have a satiny, buttery pudding that will make grandma's secret recipe look like a knockoff. Only simple ingredients, including nonhydrogenated coconut oil, Dutch cocoa powder, dehydrated raw cane juice, and vanilla. Available in Chocolate and Vanilla (morinu.com).

Chocolate Chips

Move over, Toll House. Mama had to move on to something veg!

Swap that ⟳⟳⟳⟳

Nestlé Toll House Semi-Sweet Chocolate Morsels

⟳⟳⟳⟳ *for this*

Sunspire Organic Chocolate and Carob Chips

Sunspire's chocolate and carob chips are sweetened with malted barley and corn, with no refined sugars (obviously). They also offer Fair Trade Cacao Chips made with organic chocolate and flavorings (sunspire.com).

Swap that ⟳⟳⟳⟳

Hershey's Premier White Chips

⟳⟳⟳⟳ *for this*

VeganSweets White Chocolate Chips

They may be dairy-free, but they are no less smooth and creamy. Made with palm oil, cocoa butter, soy, and vanillin (veganstore.com).

Sprinkles

Swap that ⟿

⟿ *for this*

Let's Do . . . Sprinkelz Organic Sprinkles

It's just not cool to deprive a kid of sprinkles. Let's Do makes desserts festive without nasty chemical dyes or fake ingredients. Available in Confetti, Chocolatey, and Carnival (edwardandsons.com).

Agar Agar

A substitute for gelatin, agar agar is a thickener used to increase the viscosity of soups, jellies, and desserts. How are the two different? Agar agar is made from sea vegetable flakes; gelatin is derived from the collagen in the skin and bones and sometimes the intestines of cows and horsies. Any questions?

Eden Agar Agar Flakes

An all-purpose gelatin alternative, these flakes are made from a medley of eight wild sea veggies and aren't whitened or deodorized by artificial dyes or bleaches. They make a damn good pudding and are low in sodium, calories, and fat and free of any cholesterol (edenfoods.com).

Chia Seeds

Remember those freakish chia pet commercials? Well, chia is back in a big vegan way. Chia seeds have become popular in vegan baking to bind ingredients. Just grind them up and mix with water, and you get a gooey material that sticks everything together when heated. They can be used as an egg substitute for cakes, cookies, and brownies as well as for making veggie burger patties, "meatloaf," and "meatballs." If you're making a light-colored dessert, make sure to buy the white seeds; otherwise you'll end up with a funky-looking cake. Look for organic chia seeds at your local health-food store or online at nutiva.com.

Shortening

Many baking recipes call for shortening to get that crispy or flaky texture, but it's some bad stuff. Vegetable shortening (like Crisco) is often made with partially hydrogenated oils, which contain trans fat. But shortening can also come from the fat or lard of an animal. Barf. If you must bake with it, stick with brands that ditch the trans fat and use better ingredients.

Spectrum's shortening is nonhydrogenated and made with 100 percent organic expeller-pressed palm oil (spectrumorganics.com).

Condensed Milk and Cream

Swap that 〜〜〜〜

Eagle Brand Sweetened Condensed Milk

〜〜〜〜 *for this*

*Soymilke Condensed Soymilk

This is a miracle product for me. It's GMO- and gluten-free and is ideal for making gooey sheet brownies, pumpkin pie, and blondie bars. The palm oil in Soymilke's vegan milk is sourced from Brazil, so it doesn't affect the orangutan habitat (look it up, sister; olvebra.com).

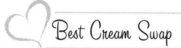 *Best Cream Swap*

*MimicCreme Cream Substitute

Swap out dairy cream for this vegan soy- and gluten-free substitute. Great for sauces, confections, gravies, cakes, hot chocolate (yum!), and coffee. One-quart containers available in Unsweetened, Sweetened, and Sugar-Free Sweetened (mimiccreme.com).

Marshmallows

How in the hell are we expected to live without s'mores? Huh?! Someone please tell me. Thanks to a few passionate brands, we can have our gelatin-free marshmallows and eat them too.

Swap that ⟋⟋⟋⟋

Kraft Marshmallows

⟋⟋⟋⟋ for this

*Chicago Soydairy Dandies Vegan Marshmallows

Fluffy and light just like conventional marshmallows, Dandies even get that crispy, burned outside when you roast them over a fire. Bonus: they're gluten-free (chicagosoydairy.com).

Sweet & Sara Vegan Marshmallows

Created by a vegan who couldn't stand living without her favorite childhood snack, the rice crispy treat, Sweet & Sara brings variety. Though it's tough for me to choose between Dandies and Sweet & Sara marshmallows, these are much puffier. The company has introduced gummy mallows in a handful of flavors alongside s'mores, rice crispy treats, macaroons, and biscotti. Marshmallows available in traditional Vanilla, Toasted Coconut, Strawberry, Cinnamon Pecan, and Minis (sweetandsara.com).

KIM'S PICK: Sweet & Sara Minis for your winter cups of hot cocoa.

Swap that ⟳⟳⟳⟳

Marshmallow Fluff

⟳⟳⟳⟳ *for this*

*Suzanne's Specialties Ricemellow Creme

I grew up on Fluffernutters, and even though they aren't the healthiest thing on the planet (not even close), they are one tasty comfort treat. If you don't know what the hell I'm talking about, you are deprived. It's two pieces of bread sandwiching peanut butter and marshmallow creme. Replace the traditional Marshmallow Fluff, which contains egg whites, with this gluten-free jar of fun. You'll want to eat it out of the jar (suzannes-specialties.com).

Whipped Cream

Swap that ⟳⟳⟳⟳

Reddi-wip Whipped Cream

⟳⟳⟳⟳ *for this*

Soyatoo Soy Whip and Rice Whip

I was pleasantly surprised when I pressed that nozzle and saw fluffy white swirls of whipped cream land atop my hot chocolate. I'm not crazy about the flavor alone—it's not bad; it just takes some getting used to. I just don't recommend spraying it in your mouth point-blank like you did when you were a kid (soyatoo.com).

Beverage Swaps

Tea

Anyone who knows me will tell you that I have a slight infatuation with tea. Some might call it a problem. Every time I go to the grocery store, I buy another flavor, even though I have a pantry full of tea at home. But there are worse addictions. Tea is packed with antioxidants, and it helps your body detoxify, supports healthy immune and digestive systems, and fights bad cholesterol. Here are some of my favorite brands. Some are medicinal, some help you sleep, and others are just plain heartwarming.

Yogi Tea

Yogi allows you to get creative, with a tea that fits every mood, purpose, or story. All of the teas are made with hand-selected herbs, spices, and ingredients from around the globe. There are too many to name, but some highlights are Bedtime (promotes restful sleep), Breathe Deep (supports clear breathing), Chai Green (energizing), and Echinacea Immune Support (supports immune function). Yogi even created a line of Woman's Teas, which targets all of our freakish womanly issues, pregnancy, and that time of the month (yogiproducts.com).

Numi Organic Tea

Pure, exotic teas that inspire overall well-being. Eighty percent of the raw ingredients Numi sources are certified fair trade. Choose from Jasmine Green, White Rose, Orange Spice, Golden Chai, Breakfast Blend, Chamomile Lemon, Rooibos Chai, Decaf Black Vanilla, and White Nectar (numitea.com).

Tazo Teas

Tazo offers a rich variety of loose-leaf teas hand-made in small batches so they stay nice and fresh. And don't worry about getting your hands on them—they're available at Starbucks. Available in Decaf Lotus Green Tea, Green Ginger, Zen Green Tea, Decaf Tazo Chai, Organic Darjeeling, Awake Tea, China Green Tips, Green Ginger, and Earl Grey (tazo.com).

Good Earth Teas

Soothing, herbal teas made on American soil. Choose from teas in Red, Superfruit, Green, Chai, Black, White, Organic, and Medicinal (goodearthteas.com).

KIM'S PICKS: Organic Seven Spice Chai Tea, Organic Green Tea with Mango, Peach and Pineapple, Organic Jasmine Blossom Green Tea, Decaf White Tea, and English Breakfast.

Zhena's Gypsy Tea

A collection of premium organic, fair-trade, 100 percent natural teas brought to you by a true gypsy and kick-ass woman and mother. Zhena started selling her teas more than a decade ago to raise money for surgeries that meant the survival of her newborn son. Now with a healthy son in tow, Zhena has also given birth to a global tea brand that gives back to the community. Zhena's offers tea sachets, loose-leafs, and seasonal sips for every mood (gypsytea.com).

KIM'S PICK: Coconut Chai.

Soda

Every now and then, we get tired of being the good girl. We want to indulge in something that makes us feel cheap and mediocre—a nice, cold caffeinated soda. Aw, just like those good ole summers when you used to let the neighborhood boys look up your skirt for a quarter. But here's the thing: you can have a soda without feeling like a closet freak. Here are a few that I keep around for emergencies or when I want to change things up.

Remember darlin' . . . everything in moderation, and you won't be like the rest of the nation. Capeesh?

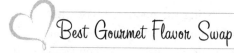

Best Transition Soda

Swap that

Canned Soda

for this

Zevia All Natural Soda

Zero calories. Zero artificial ingredients or colors. Zero to little sodium. And 100 percent natural flavor. Zevia is sweetened with stevia (a healthy, plant-based sweetener) and tastes just as lovely as the stuff that wrecks your body. Available in six-packs at every major grocer. The purchase feels no different either. Choose from Orange, Cola, Caffeine Free Cola, Ginger Root Beer, Ginger Ale, Grapefruit Citrus, Lemon Lime Twist, Grape, Cream, Mountain Zevia, and Black Cherry (zevia.com).

Best Gourmet Flavor Swap

Dry Soda

If soda companies were rated like restaurants, Dry Soda would be a Michelin Five-Star. Its gourmet natural sodas are flavored with fruit, flower, and herb extracts and come in a sleek and chic glass bottle. Sweetened with a small dose of pure cane sugar and just the right amount of carbonation, they contain no more than four ingredients in every bottle. Simple but not overly sweet, and only 45 to 70 calories in every flavor. Choose from Cucumber, Vanilla Bean, Juniper Berry, Lavender, Lemongrass, Blood Orange, and Rhubarb (drysoda.com).

KIM'S PICK: Lavender. You'll never want to pick up a Coca Cola again.

Izze Sparkling Juice

Give it up for Izze. My favorite in this group, Izze contains pure fruit juice, no caffeine or preservatives, and nothin' artificial. Each sparkling soda is low in calories and available at every darn retailer and café you can think of. The company now also carries Izze Fortified, which is juiced up with niacin and vitamins C and B-6. Choose from Pomegranate, Grapefruit, Lime, Blueberry, Clementine, Peach, Apple, and Blackberry (izze.com).

KIM'S PICK: Clementine, which is citrusy, fresh, and perfect for a hot summer day.

Hot Lips Soda

The savvy packaging got me, but the taste is what did me in. Just real fruit soda pop filtered with pure cane sugar and organic lemon juice. No corn syrup, artificial flavors, or concentrates. The company also cares about the earth—80 percent of the bottles are made from recycled glass (hotlipssoda.com).

Wine

I'm not a big drinker—in fact, I've never liked the taste of alcohol—but I have plenty of friends who are winos and proud of it. Now, there are couple megadowners when it comes to traditional wines, and one might throw you for a loop. Sadly, most wines aren't vegan (gasp!). A handful of animal ingredients can go into the winemaking process. The most common are isinglass (a pure form of gelatin that comes from fish bladders), gelatin (an extract that comes from boiled hooves and barnyard body parts), egg whites, and casein (a protein found in most cow's milk). Sick, huh?

Second, nobody would argue about the morning after. Hangovers blow. You hit the town feeling like Carrie Bradshaw and wake up with a sandpaper tongue, a phone number scribbled on your thigh, and a slight inkling that you mass-"sexted" in search of a booty call. If this sounds like your Friday night—or, even worse, your Tuesday night—organic wines are where it's at.

Organic wines are full-bodied, sophisticated, and lower in sugar and sulfites—sulfites are the very culprit that has you eating Excedrin like candy. Organic varieties still contain sulfites, but they are added in excess to conventional wines as a preservative. And hello?! No pesticides. Recall that wine comes from grapes, which are sprayed just like any other fruit or veggie. Here are a few great vegan and healthy swaps for traditional wines.

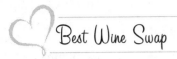
Best Wine Swap

Frey Organic Wines

This Mendocino County winery is family owned and recognized as being America's first certified organic winery. There are no added sulfites in its wines, which allows you to enjoy the distinct, natural flavors. Frey also took home the 2003 Veggie Award from *VegNews* as the best vegan wine. For its white wines, it uses bentonite clay as the fining agent rather than the typical animal ingredients. I serve it at every dinner party, and everyone ends up writing down the name before they leave (freywine.com).

Bonterra Organic Wines, White Wines

Though Bonterra uses egg whites in the fining of the red wines, no animal ingredients are used in the production process for white wines (bonterra.com).

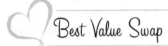
Best Value Swap

Orleans Hill Wines

Crisp, youthful wines made from grapes grown organically on the outskirts of Nevada City, California. And they're affordable to boot ($10 and under). The entire line is vegan-friendly (chartrandimports.com).

Albet i Noya Petit Albet Organic Wines

This winery estate in Spain has converted all 187 acres of vineyards over to organic farming methods, and it sources all the grapes from local organic farmers (albetinoya.com).

Coturri Wines

Straight from California's renowned wine country, Sonoma County, Coturri hand-bottles organic wines with no inoculation with sulfites or yeast cultures and no added water, acids, or concentrates that may screw up the way nature made them. Coturri doesn't broadcast that its wines are vegan-friendly, but they are (coturriwinery.com).

For more vegan wine options, check out barnivore.com/wine.

Beer

You probably owe the extra fifteen pounds you gained freshman year of college to beer. After all, a party wasn't a party without a keg and a beer bong, right? But, beer doesn't have to be all that bad. On the good side, it's fat-free, low in sugar, and high in fiber and contains hefty amounts of magnesium, selenium, potassium, biotin, and B vitamins. It's also known to reduce stress and lower your chances of heart disease—again, when you're not throwing back cans like a Chicago Bears fan on Super Bowl Sunday.

Now for the not so hot facts. Even though beer contains no sugar, the alcohol affects your blood-sugar levels, causing them to spike and drop. This, ladies, stimulates your appetite. And now you know why the Domino's delivery dude knows you by your nickname.

There's another major kick in the ass about beer: alcoholic drinks aren't required to disclose their ingredients or those that were used during pro-

Before you start sucking down bottles of wine like Evian, get this: up to 240 different chemicals go into the making of traditional wines, and grapes are the most pesticide-laden produce on the lot. Organic, anybody?

cessing on the packaging. So if the beer doesn't directly state it's suitable for vegans, then you have to take a lucky guess. But Skinny Bitches don't guess—they get answers, dammit. The predicament we face with the everyday brewski is quite similar to that with wine—isinglass, otherwise known as "fish bladders," is often used as a fining agent to collect yeast extract from beer. Beer crafters may also use gelatin, casein, egg whites, or chitosan (crustaceans) to get the cloudy crap from the keg.

But do not fret, my pet. There are many beer manufacturers that use vegan means to extract sediment, or they just do it the ole-fashioned way and let it settle at the bottom. How about that?

New Belgium Mothership Wit Organic Wheat Beer

Toxin-free, organic beer made from wheat and barley that was grown using sustainable farming methods. Organic bitter orange peels, coriander, and lemon peels boost the citrusy flavor (newbelgium.com).

Mt. Shasta Brewing Weed Ales and Lagers

Handcrafted ales and lagers brewed with pure, magical Mt. Shasta spring water (weedales.com).

Vegan Beers You Will Recognize

Amstel · Corona · Dos Equis · Sapporo · Heineken · Sierra Nevada · Mickey's · Miller · Coors · Rolling Rock · Tecate

For more information on vegan beers, check out barnivore.com/beer.

*Magic Hat Beers

This Vermont microbrewery brews four year-round beers and some seasonals, with gluten- and wheat-free options (magichat.net).

Redhook Beer

A collection of smooth, clean ales brewed with the highest-quality ingredients and water from the Cascade Mountains (redhook.com).

Moosehead Lager

This Canadian independent brewery has been around longer than most of our presidents. It offers a smooth, refreshing line of light and full-bodied lagers (moosehead.ca).

An asterisk (*) means the product is gluten-free.

Index

Scan this code to access bonus materials for *Skinny Bitch Book of Vegan Swaps* and other healthy living books and information.

You can also text keyword SKINNY to READIT (732348) to be sent a link to the mobile website.